WITH THE AMERICAN AMBULANCE IN FRANCE

BY
DR. JAMES R. JUDD

SICPRESS 2013
METHUEN, MASS.

Dr. James R. Judd's *With the American Ambulance in France* was originally published in 1919 by the Honolulu Star-Bulletin Press.

©2013, SicPress.com

14 Pleasant St.

Methuen, Massachusetts.

sales@sicpress.com

TABLE OF CONTENTS

PREFACE

Spread over the battlefield of the Marne are numerous graves marked with white crosses and tiny tri-color flags. Late one fall afternoon in 1915 a peasant woman leading a little child by the hand was seen wandering from grave to grave and reading the names inscribed on the little white crosses. They were looking for the grave of their soldier husband and father who had died for his country and for us and our civilization. This picture has ever remained vivid in my mind.

What is to become of the fatherless children of France? Should not we Americans show our appreciation of the sacrifices made by the noble French fathers by helping to care for their children and so help rebuild the nation?

This little book was written with the idea that the entire profits of its sale will go to help the fatherless children of France. The material is based on stories told by wounded in our care and on experiences as recorded in home letters during the period from July 1915 to October 1916 when the writer and his wife had the great privilege of living with the poilus and playing a small part in the great struggle for freedom.

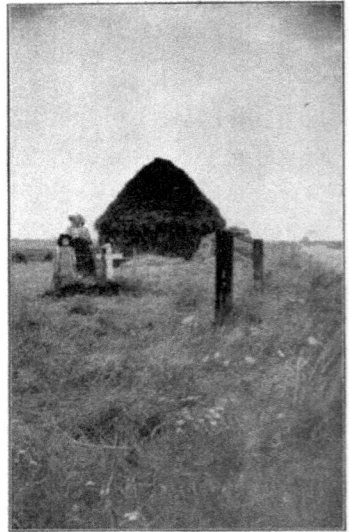

Chapter I.

Honolulu to France.

When the great war began in August, 1914, there were several hundred Americans in Paris. Many of them were tourists, visiting Paris as part of the grand tour of the continent. The others belonged to the so-called American colony and because of their long residence there considered Paris their home.

When the Germans hacked their way through Belgium and the vast horde of Huns streamed across the frontier toward the heart of France, carrying death and destruction in their wake, somewhat of a panic developed in Paris among those who were anxious to get away. Crowds collected in front of the banks eager to get money. Hotels and shops demanded cash payments. Paper money was discounted and gold was at a premium. Holders of large letters of credit suddenly found themselves poor. The train service was overtaxed and inadequate to handle the crowds, and automobiles were hired at fabulous prices. Trunks were left behind in the mad rush. As an illustration of the state of mind, a friend told me that an excited American rushed up to him on the street exclaiming, "Do you speak English? I will give you $500 to get me out of Paris."

The Americans divided themselves into two classes. First, there were those who were part of the crowd of fugitives and resorted to every means in their power in order to effect their escape. The others were those who, loyal to the dictates of their moral obligation, resolved to stay to the last extremity and aid the city they loved.

Among these last there was fortunately an organization comprising the American Hospital of Paris, an admirable institution, which for several years past had been maintained by Americans. With the American Hospital as a basis of unity the American Ambulance was founded and its services were offered to the French government.

On the third day of September, when the Germans were at Compiègne, barely 50 miles away, the French government moved to Bordeaux. The Americans were released from their promised service, leaving them free to escape from the investment of Paris which, at that time, seemed inevitable. To the eternal honor of our fellow countrymen be it remembered that they refused to accept the release from their promise and decided to cast their lot and if necessary risk their lives with the people of Paris. Then came the battle of the Marne and Paris was saved. From a small beginning the Ambulance grew to an organization caring for over 1500 wounded a day and maintaining more than 300 ambulances on duty in Paris and at the front. The cost of maintaining this work has been borne entirely by the American people.

It is difficult to estimate the value of the work of the American Ambulance in this war. No less important than the material aid rendered the French wounded has been the moral effect of the organization of cultivating and maintaining a friendly feeling for America and every worker in the Ambulance—doctor, nurse and ambulance driver—on returning to America has been an ardent proselyte, burning with a sense of righteousness of the cause of the Allies and eager for the United States to take her proper place in the struggle.

It was to join this organization that we started for France on June 12, 1915, and a few weeks later we found ourselves aboard the steamship "St. Louis" leaving New York harbor. A little crowd of friends was at the wharf to say farewell, but there was no band or "leis."

The "St. Louis" was an old ship, steady in smooth weather, but not over clean or comfortable. The label "American Line" was painted in huge white letters on the ship's sides. At night a cluster of electric lights with a reflector was lowered over each side and so placed that the letters were well illuminated. The ship was crowded. Since the war the American line has come into sudden popularity and consequently the rates have risen. We had a deck stateroom for which we paid $300 plus a $10 war tax. The bath was a tiny affair and a long ways off in the bowels of the ship. The sanitary arrangements left much to be desired. The food was fairly good. There was an orchestra of five pieces which played during meal time. Altogether we got on quite well and had, no kick coming, provided the old tub landed us safely at Liverpool. We had provided ourselves with life preserver jackets in New York and kept them handy. The last night out, as we were in the danger zone, many of the passengers camped out on deck and talked most of the night.

On July 19th land appeared and at eight o'clock in the evening we sailed up the Mersey and were docked at Liverpool. While it was still light, we lined up in the saloon, our passports were inspected and stamped by a benevolent looking old gentleman and we climbed off the St. Louis, grateful that our voyage was safely over.

Liverpool looked as grimy and unattractive as usual. It was Sunday night and everything was quiet. There were no signs of war. We managed to lay in a supply of newspapers, fruit and candy and an hour or so before midnight we started on a special steamer train for London. We sped through the dark night at a great rate of speed and could not help contrasting the superiority of the English railroad travel over that of the United States. There were no sudden stops and jerks such as one encounters unexpectedly anywhere from San Francisco to New York. The towns we passed through were dimly lighted on account of Zeppelins. The curtains of our train were drawn so that the light did not shine out. At half past three in the morning we reached Euston station and a great scramble for luggage ensued. Finally we extricated our baggage, piled it on a "four wheeler" and hied ourselves to the Savoy Hotel. At the hotel two pieces of baggage were found to be missing, so I dashed back to the station in a taxi and found the two bags safely reposing on the platform just where we had left them. The station was now full of sailors who had arrived there just after us. As I started back to the Savoy several sailors tried to hail my taxi, so I stopped and told them to "pile in." The taxi was rapidly filled to its capacity, and those who couldn't find room on the seats, sat on the steps and mud-guards. A much whiskered tar, smelling of salt water and tobacco, was my seat companion. He said that they were sailors of the North Sea fleet and were crossing London to Victoria station on their way to Portsmouth, he thought. Patrolling the North Sea was bitterly cold work and they were longing for the German fleet to come out. It was then broad daylight and we passed several dignified bobbies who yelled at the sailors to get off the running boards, to which the tars responded in true democratic fashion by applying their thumbs to their noses and actively wiggling their fingers.

London seemed very much the same as on previous visits and gave one the same comfortable and home-like feeling. There was a little less street traffic and fewer American tourists were in evidence. A good many uniforms were to be seen on the streets, and huge posters and notices calling for enlistments were prominently displayed. There were recruiting stations here and there, but we saw few recruits. We hunted up our favorite restaurant, the "Cheshire Cheese," and enjoyed a delicious dinner of sole, chops, pigeon pie, peas and toasted cheese. At the "Empire" afterwards we saw a mediocre performance before a crowded house, with orchestra seats at 10s apiece.

At the French consulate hundreds of people were ahead of us waiting to get their papers. The work was so heavy that an adjoining residence was used to handle the crowd. Finally after several hours waiting we received tickets from the porter and when our numbers were called we were allowed to enter a large living room already filled with all kinds of people. Women and children composed the majority of those waiting and all looked very weary. Finally the numbers are called again and we proceeded upstairs to a room where several officials were seated at small tables. In turn each one of us was seated at a table facing an official and subjected to an inquiry as to the reasons for wishing to go to France. I showed several letters which produced little effect until letters from Dr. Marques, French Consul of Honolulu, stating in French the object of our journey, were read. These letters were like magic and our passports were given us without further trouble.

At ten the next morning we left London for Folkestone. The usual charming views of rural England were changed by seeing here and there training camps and bodies of troops drilling in the fields. Aside from that it was hard to tell that this mighty nation was at war. At Folkestone we formed in line, passed through a docket and our papers were examined and stamped. We were then allowed to proceed aboard the channel steamer "Sussex." No staterooms were to be had, so we procured steamer chairs and prepared for the worst of our four and a half hours trip to Dieppe. There were many vessels to be seen in the channel as we left the English shore and several destroyers gave us a feeling of security. Soon we passed out of sight of land, ships and destroyers and were alone. There was quite a sea and the spray splashed over us sitting out on deck. The weather was surprisingly cold and chilly. The steamer was crowded with passengers, most of them seasick, and they were not always particular to get to leeward when they had to pay tribute to Neptune. I remember seeing a little French cabin-boy or "mousse" trying to persuade a disconsolate looking English boy that it was desirable to pass his fingers down his throat. This pantomime continued for some time, but the English lad either would not be persuaded or felt too badly to attempt it.

The cold gray water of the channel looked very uninviting. We wondered if there were any German submarines around and if this part of the channel was protected by a steel net. We were all subject to a feeling of helplessness as we had at least expected an escort. That our fears were not groundless was shown by subsequent events when the "Sussex" was torpedoed, and this act of barbarism became an international question.

A trip never seemed so slow, until finally we feasted our eyes on the white cliffs of Dieppe, which looked so much like those we had left at Folkestone, as if the land had been cleft and pushed apart.

At Dieppe there was the animation and vivacity of conversation that one finds in a French seaport town. Once again we were herded into line and our papers examined and stamped. But nothing mattered now. We were on the beloved soil of France again.

A surprisingly good train carried us to Paris in three hours. While we enjoyed an excellent table d'hôte dinner for five francs, we looked out of the car windows at the peaceful Normandy country and could not realize that the most terrible warfare the world has ever seen was in progress a few miles away.

At the Paris station we were delighted to find that our baggage had come through with us, and taking it along in our fiacre we were soon comfortably settled at the splendid Edouard VII hotel.

Chapter II.

Paris.

How thrilling, almost magical after a good sleep to wake up in Paris, stroll out on the boulevards, rub one's eyes and realize that we are really there! The weather was delightful for midsummer, a temperature of 70° with clear sunny skies. Beautiful flowers were grouped for sale at the street corners. We recognized our old friends the Opera, Café de la Paix, the Madeleine and the Place de la Concorde at the end of the rue Royale.

Even in Paris it is hard to realize that war is at hand. There are soldiers to be seen here and there. Some of them are crippled, walking with crutches or have bandages on their heads. There are a good many women in mourning. Nearly all the shops are open and the larger magasins like the Lafayette and Printemps, are crowded with shoppers. The restaurants are well filled with patrons and there is the same long menu of delicious food with apparently little elevation of prices. We noticed only that the Grand Vatel and Tour d'Argent are closed. The Louvre is closed but a part of the Luxemburg is open, also the Musée Carnavalet. The big, noisy busses are no more. This is not a matter of regret as they are doing useful work at the front transporting troops. Women do men's work as conductors on the trains and metro, driving fiacres and cleaning streets. I have never seen the streets of Paris so clean. The banks close from twelve to two on account of the lack of employees and many of the stores do the same. There are crowds of people sitting out on the sidewalks of the cafes in the delightful Paris fashion. At ten o'clock the cafés close and no music is allowed in any restaurants.

At night one notices a great difference from the Paris of peace times. The night life of Montmartre is no more. The Bal Bouiller, Moulin Rouge and other places from which Americans have gained erroneous ideas of French life and character , are closed. The streets are quite dark but not as dark as we found them in London. The darkening of the streets is for two reasons. First as a precaution against Zeppelin raids, and second, as a matter of economy. Most of the theatres are running, but grand opera will not be attempted. On a Sunday afternoon we had a four hours' musical treat at the Opéra Comique. Charpentier's "Louise" was given admirably. The house was crowded, many of the audience being soldiers and some of them convalescents with their arms in slings or their heads bandaged. It was pathetic to see a number of blind soldiers in the audience. At the end of the performance Madame Chenal sang the soul-stirring "Marseillaise" with the audience standing. We could feel thrills run up and down our backs.

Although music is forbidden in cafés and restaurants, yet the government thinks that good music is a beneficial tonic for the people, and there are fine concerts in the Tuilleries and Luxembourg gardens. Soldiers attend these concerts in large numbers and the music receives much appreciation as shown by the attention and applause.

On bright sunny afternoons we enjoyed sitting out on the sidewalk of the Café de la Paix and watching the crowds pass by. War does not prevent the Parisians from enjoying this pleasure, and although there are many uniforms and some mutilés to be seen, it is hard to realize that men are being killed barely fifty miles away.

With all the losses and suffering France has endured there is no depression, but a smiling philosophical attitude is apparent on all sides. Truly it takes a war to show a nation's real character.

We heard an interesting spy story the other day. A French girl who had lived in Alsace and knew the German language stepped on a man's foot as she was entering the Metro. The man was dressed as an English officer and to her surprise he swore a German oath. She resolved to follow him, so got off when he did and reported him to a gendarme, who shrugged his shoulders and wouldn't do anything. She then followed him to a house and noting the address, sped to the nearest police station. The house was quickly raided and not only was the spurious English officer caught but two other spies and a quantity of incriminating papers.

Germany had the most complete spy system the world has ever seen. Not only was Paris well covered but the country towns and villages as well. The authorities have warned the people to be on their guard by attaching notices in public places "Taisez-vous, Méfiez-vous. Les oreilles d'ennemis vous écoutent." This warning was not taken very seriously and was a favorite theme for jest at the theatres.

One of the chief topics of conversation is, "When will the war end?" Great things are always expected of the offensive "next year," after the bad winter weather is over. There is some talk of the pinch of starvation in Germany and the possibilities of a revolution. It seems that thinking people do not take much stock in these ideas.

The starvation of Germany is counter-balanced by Germany's food economies and her increased agricultural acquisitions in Belgium, Northern France, Poland and Servia. Thousands of prisoners furnish much of the agricultural labor. A revolution is discredited because the great mass of the German people have been taught and trained that the government should do their thinking for them. No, the war will be brought to an end by military superiority, and that means a long and bloody conflict. The battle of the Marne saved Paris, saved France, saved civilization. The noble Belgian defense, the heroism of the French soldier and "the contemptible little British army" at the battle of the Marne crumpled up Germany's plan of world conquest right at the start. But without England's aid France would have been paralyzed with most of her coal and iron mines in the hands of the enemy. After the battle of the Marne France's task was stupendous—to hold back the long battle line until British troops could be trained and take over a powerful position. This could never have been accomplished without the superiority of the British navy.

Germany launched a tremendous attack at Verdun, planning to beat her way through by main force. Those weeks and months of struggle were anxious days in France. When news of the terrible slaughter became generally known, there were questions among the civilians: "Why don't they give up Verdun and let the Germans have it? It isn't worth all the slaughter." "No," the French soldier said "Ils ne passeront pas." "Why don't the English start an offensive to relieve the pressure on Verdun?" "Don't you know the English are not ready yet and they are carrying out Joffre's plan? They will attack when the right time comes." We often thought that the idea that the French were being sacrificed at Verdun, while the British were inactive was part of the subtle German propaganda.

We kept wondering what the United States was going to. do in this great world mix-up. We came to France with the idea that this was a European war, the breaking of treaties and invasion of territory, far apart from America. We were not long in France before we discovered that the Allies were fighting for the very principles on which the foundations of our liberty rest and that there could be no such thing as neutrality of heart. A German victory in Europe meant America as the next victim in the world conquest. The Americans whom we have talked with think that our country has played an ignoble part thus far. We have made money out of the war, lots of it, and have sent back very little in comparison to our gains. But there is a feeling of confidence that the time will come when America will see that the Allies are fighting our battles and that the United States will take her place in the struggle for democracy.

Chapter III.

The American Ambulance of Neuilly-sur-Seine.

Going up the Champs Elysées, past the Arc de Triomphe and along the Avenue des Grandes Armées one comes to the Porte Maillot. Passing through this gate one enters the suburb of Neuilly and is now officially out of Paris. As the taxi drivers can claim an extra rate of fare after passing through the gate, we used to pay off the driver at the gate, walk through and take another taxi to drive to the Ambulance. That was in the early days. Later on we learned to economize by going on the tram or metro for 30 centimes.

At the beginning of the war a splendid new school building, the Lycée Pasteur, was reaching completion. The Board of Governors of the American Hospital in Paris offered to the French government to maintain a hospital for the care of wounded soldiers for the duration of the war, and this building was assigned to them. It should not be forgotten that in the war of 1870 the Americans of Paris organized and maintained an American ambulance which rendered valuable service.

By completing the equipment and installing the necessary hospital furniture, it was found that the Lycée Pasteur lended itself admirably for the purpose of a hospital. The construction of the building with plenty of windows, splendid lighting and ventilation rendered it an ideal hospital building, and it is doubtful if among the 4,000 or more war hospitals in France, there is a finer institution. There are accommodations for 600 patients in round numbers with large wards and small wards for officers and special cases. A number of the wards are maintained by contributions from different cities and states, and this fact is designated by names over the doorways——New York, Boston, Philadelphia, Chicago, Virginia, Rhode Island and others are there. We hope there will be a "Hawaii Ward" some day.

The Ambulance Committee consists of:
Capt. Frank H. Mason, Chairman.
Robert Bacon.
Lawrence V. Benét.
Dr. C. W. Du Bouchet.
F. W. Monahan.
L. V. Twyeffort.
Mrs. W. K. Vanderbilt.
Mrs. H. P. Whitney.

The surgical staff of about thirty doctors are almost all volunteers from America, and some of our most famous surgeons have served there. Among them are Drs. Blake, Hutchinson, Harte, Powers, Murphy, Cushing and Crile.

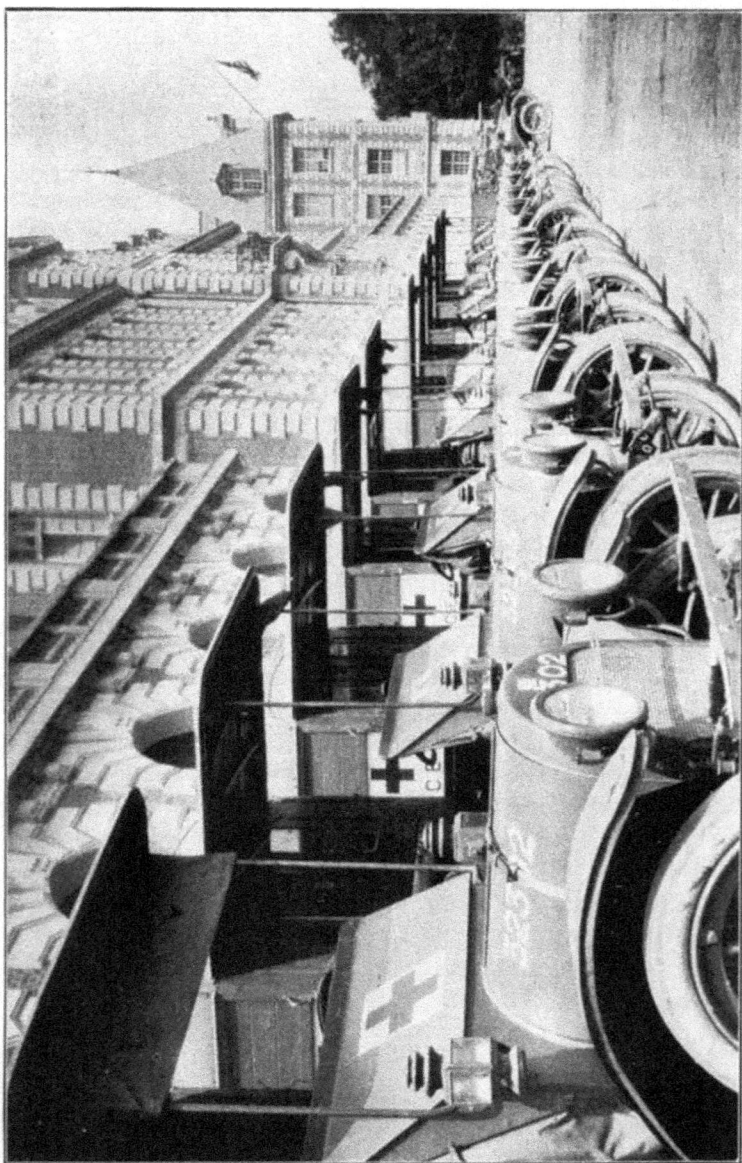

Automobiles ready to go to the railroad station for wounded.

The dental department, organized by Dr. Hayes and ably conducted by volunteer American dentists, has done splendid work, especially in restoration of shattered jaws.

The nursing staff consists of about 90 trained nurses, most of whom have come from America. There are a large number of auxiliary nurses under the able direction of Mrs. George Munroe.

The orderly work is done by volunteers, business men, artists, dilitantes, Rhodes scholars from Oxford and others.

A useful feature of the ambulance is the transportation service. A large number of cars are ready day or night to go the Gare la Chapelle, receive loads of wounded and transport them to hospitals designated by. the authorities.

The Field Service sections stationed at different parts of the front render valuable service to the French and have transported over 400,000 wounded. This part of the ambulance service is ably directed by A. Piatt Andrew, formerly assistant treasurer of the United States.

On my first visit to the hospital. I hunted up my former teacher, Dr. Blake, and found him making "rounds." He gave me a cordial welcome and upon my asking for work, said that there was plenty of it and that he would be glad to have me join his staff.

The first sensation of a civilian doctor on starting to work in a ward of French soldiers is one of bewilderment. There is a mass of wooden frames, pulleys and weights holding shattered bones in comfortable positions. The awful looking wounds make one wonder how a man ever survived such an injury and then how will it be possible to save these shattered limbs. At once one is impressed by the courage, cheerfulness and patience of the French soldier. Some are mere peasant boys of 18 to 20, others are educated men, merchants, school teachers, law and medical students. The majority are country boys, sons of the soil. They all expect to get well and most of them do. The worst cases are kept out on porches, where they have the benefit of the fresh air and sunshine.

At present all the patients are "old cases" and the operations performed are for the removal of pieces of shell and dead splinters of bone. The patients are carefully X-rayed and the pieces of shell located. Then there is an electrical apparatus invented by Professor Bergonie of Bordeaux by means of which one can feel a piece of shell vibrating in the flesh. Even with these aids the pieces of shell are very elusive and sometimes surprisingly difficult to find. The work consists of morning rounds with Dr. Blake, afterwards operations if there are any to be done and then the dressings.

L. has been assigned to a small ward, where she makes beds, helps at the "pansements," takes temperatures and pulses, helps with the meals and in many other ways. She looks real business-like in her French Red Cross uniform and enjoys the work thoroughly.

The food served to the wounded is very good and the blessés are very appreciative of what is 'done for them. The approximate cost of maintaining the hospital is $1,000.00 a day, and this is entirely a matter of subscription.

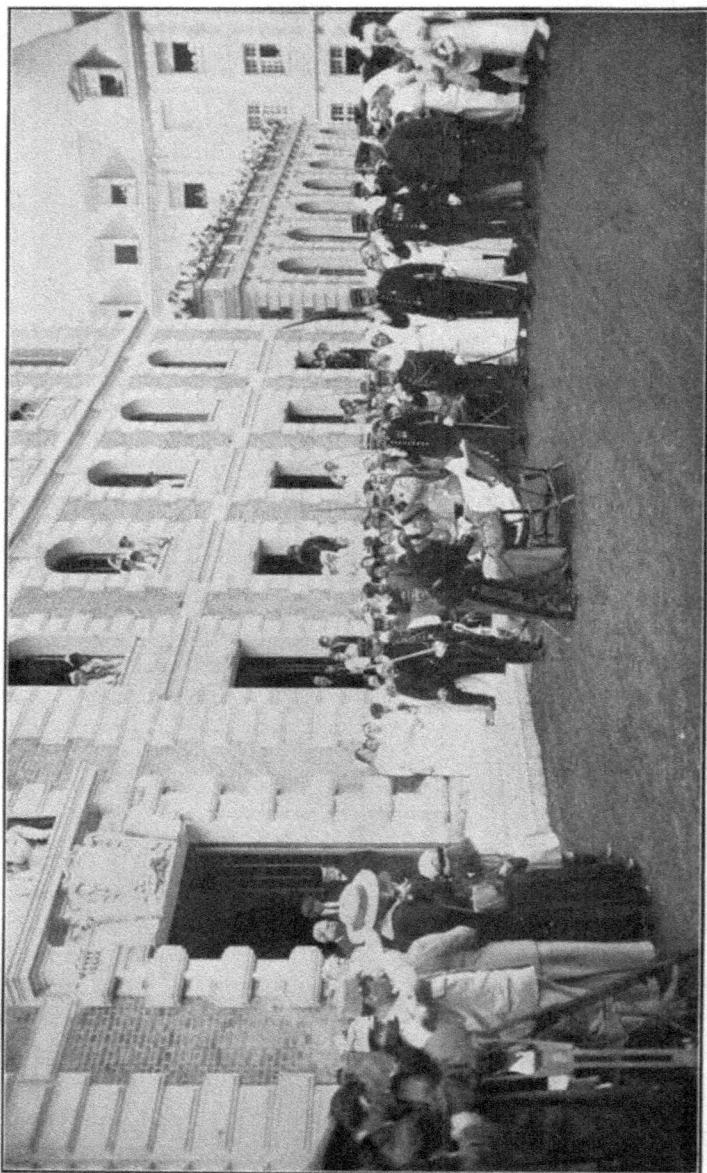

The American Ambulance at Neuilly.

In order to economize time we moved to a small villa near the hospital, kept by the head waiter of the Ritz. He is an Italian and speaks several languages and sets a good table. We have our coffee in our room at 7 a. m., and are at the hospital at 8 o'clock. We have lunch in the basement of the hospital with a crowd of 200, composed of doctors, nurses, auxiliaries, ambulance drivers and personnel and the noise is like that of a boiler factory. However, everyone seems to have a good appetite and to be in good spirits. At night we are too tired to go out, so dine at the Villa for 3 francs. For sixty cents or less, as a franc is worth about 18 cents, we have a delicious meal and the enemy barely 50 miles away. Fancy getting any such meal in New York for 60 cents I It can't be that the food itself is so much superior, but it is the art in cooking it, in which the French excel.

It's a wonder that the blessés after the terrible experiences they have been through are not more nervous. With a few exceptions they are calm and patient. One of our men lay badly wounded under a pile of dead men for thirteen hours before he was rescued. The soldiers say that the German line with its concrete fortifications and heavy artillery is too strong to break through.

One of our patients was a boy of seventeen who ran away to the army as he was too young to be called. He was recovering from a wound of the abdomen and wrote a verse of poetry for me which he entitled:

En Souvenir de ma Reconnaissance.
(Poème, Sans Prétentions)
and concluded the poem as follows:
Vers vous Américains amis si précieux
Des bons soins que dans votre hôpital j'ai reçus
Je me souviendrai durant toute ma vie
Dites-moi? Comment voulez-vous que j'oublie?
Mais je ne veux pas donner de détails menus
Ma reconnaissance vers vous s'envole
Semblable à un léger oiseau frivole.
Charmant petit oiseau, s'échappant du fond du coeur
Vous souhaitant pour toujours joie et bonheur.

In parenthesis he wrote in English: "Excuse my writing because I am in the bed."

A présent je suis sauvé et dans ce petit coin du nouveau monde transporté dans notre chère France. je suis soigné admirablement, jamais je n'oublierai le dévouement dont font preuve Infirmiers et Infirmières. Leur souvenirs restera toujours gravé dans ma mémoire. Vive la France! Vive les Américains!

A big tile-layer from Montreal responded to the call of France and is now recovering from a bad wound of the arm. He enjoys talking English and acting as interpreter for the nurses. A dapper little soldier lived several years in New Orleans, speaks perfect English and seems glad to be among Americans.

There is a Zouave in the ward who has lost a leg and hobbles around on crutches. He owns a fine setter dog which is the only animal pet of the hospital. The dog was at

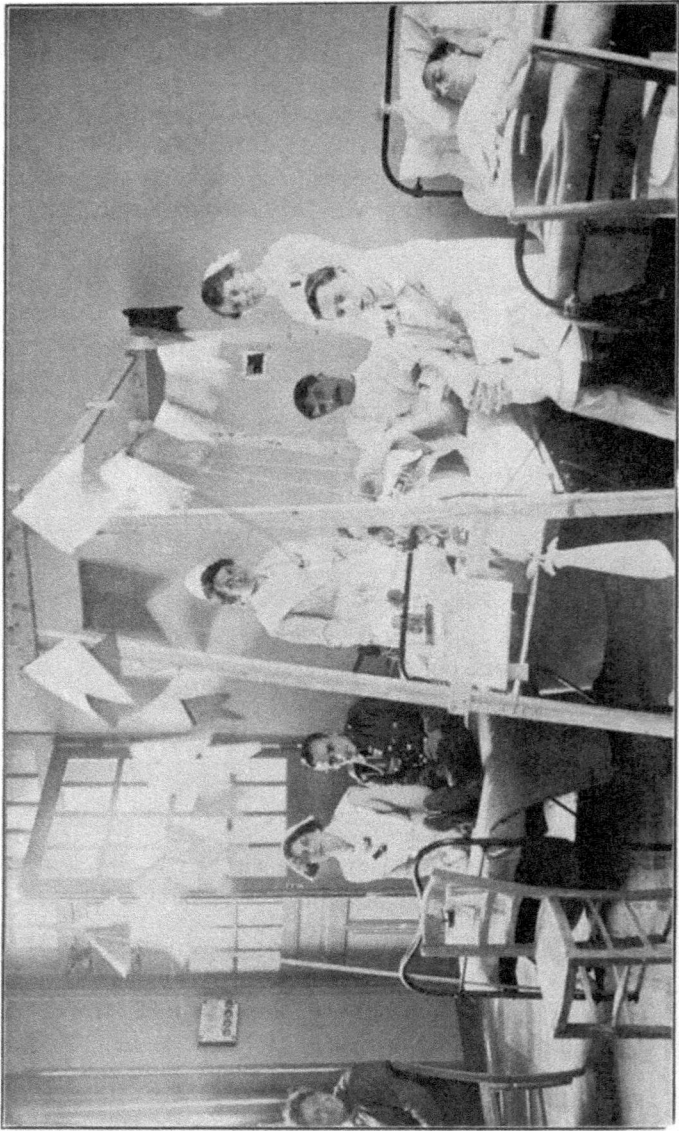

The last three British Tommies at the American Ambulance, cared for by American nurses.

the front with his master when the Germans exploded a mine under a section of trench. Fortunately the dog was somewhat in the rear in the vicinity of a field kitchen and had the opportunity of saving his master's life. As soon as the explosion occurred the setter ran up and, after digging furiously awhile, hauled the Zouave out of a pile of earth. The soldier was unconscious and had a leg badly mangled but survived his injuries. The dog became a great favorite at the hospital and when the Zouave was decorated, the setter received a special ribbon.

In the wards are three British Tommies, all that are left of the British wounded brought to the ambulance after the battle of the Aisne. One of them was in the retreat from Mons and gave me a graphic account of those terrible days.

Chapter IV.

The British Tommy's Story.

After serving nine years in India and Burma, my time expired on the third of June, 1914, leaving me three years to serve on the reserve. I was just beginning to enjoy civil life when suddenly, which everyone knows, England declared war on Germany on the fourth of August. Of course, that meant I had to be called to the colors again. I reported at my depot as soon as possible. I was equipped and sent over to France and, on about the fourteenth of August, I disembarked at Saint Nazaire. I stayed there two days then went to join my regiment in Belgium. I was not there very long before I found out it was no joke but we held our own pretty well until the twenty-sixth of August. We were at Mons at the time and were forced to retire. They were all over us. Well, we started off with the enemy at our backs and I never had such an experience in my life. The enemy was easily eight times our strength, so all we could do was to keep tracking along and they were mowing us down like sheep all the time. We were wondering why we could not retaliate and make a fight of it but all we could get from our commanders was 'keep going.' True, we had very little artillery and I am sure we would have been slaughtered had we tried to make a stand. Well, we obeyed our command. We were marching along in our sleep at times. We were doing over thirty miles some days. Of course, we were marching through the night as well. Very little rest we got. As soon as we did halt we could hardly get time for a rest before the enemy was shelling us again and we had to make another move.

About the worst part of the retirement I witnessed happened to my regiment at a place called Meaux. This was on about the seventh day, I believe it was the third of September. We had been marching all night and this was about 6 a. m. We came across what we thought was a French outpost. Our colonel questioned them and they reported "all clear" so he looked for a likely place to halt us so that we could get a little snack which we were badly in need of. At last we came across a large plot of open ground with a nullah in it. We marched into this nullah. Up to now my regiment had been very fortunate. We had just been reinforced and were about 1,200 strong. Our colonel gave us orders to pile arms and take off our equipment. In less than ten

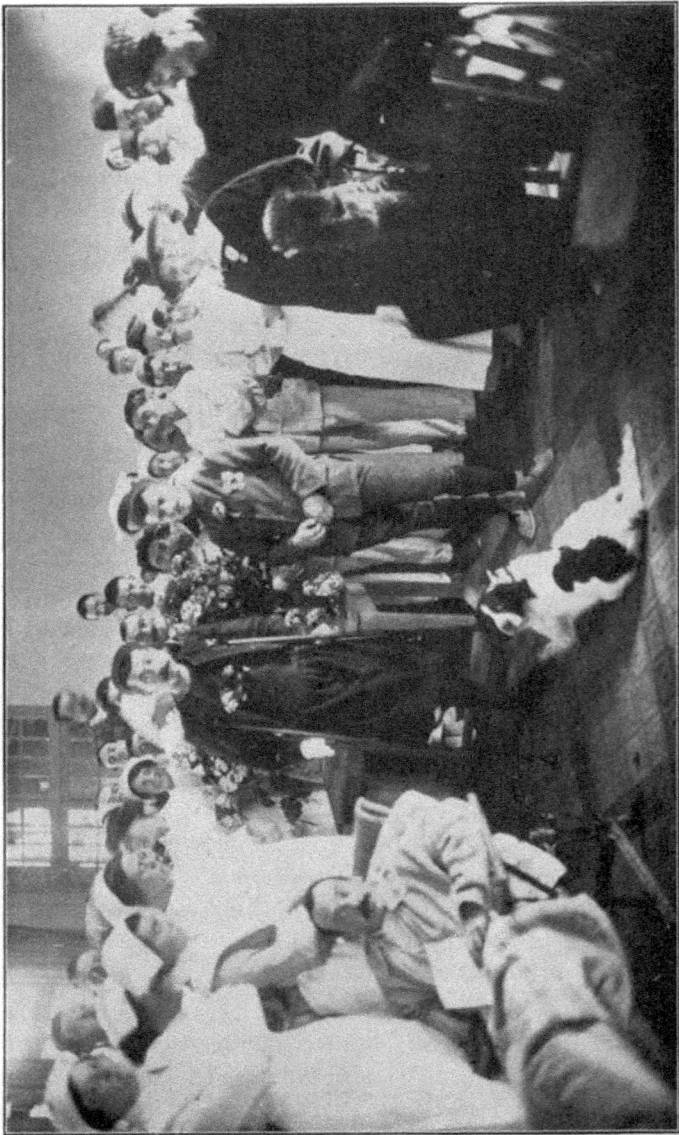

After the decoration of the Zouave and his famous dog who dug him ot of an exploded mine.

minutes after we had done so, a shower of bullets came in to us. We were surrounded by Maxims from the top of the nullah and no way out of it only to fly, which we did, most men leaving their arms behind, but not only that, we left over 700 dead and wounded, all in a few minutes. But for the Irish Fusiliers, who were on our left, we would have lost more as they kept the enemy at bay until we got under cover, when what was left of us got together again. We did not amount to 500, and there were not 200 of us armed and we also lost our Maxims. The outpost we took for French was a German outpost in French uniforms. Tricky dogs!

The next day all the brigades got together, and it was the same old thing. Retire. Retire. This was, I think, about the ninth day of it and I am sure every man in the British army was cribbing, as a soldier always does. They were all saying, "When are we going to turn around and get a smack at them?"

That night General French visited our brigade, and no doubt he visited the other brigades as well, for he must have heard about the discontent among his troops, and he said, "Men, if you will only finish this march, which you must do, it will last through the night, and tomorrow I will promise you a fight." There was not a man who did not cheer him, and every man marched all night with a good heart.

At daybreak the following morning we were seventeen miles from Paris, but little we knew that then. General French was as good as his word. We got a fight that day. We turned about and, thank God, the retreat was over. Then it became our turn. We started to advance and we gave them something for their money. We never left them alone. We would not give them time for wind. We let them see that we were made of better stuff than they were. They were surrendering by thousands, completely fagged out and we were shelling them now, mowing them down worse than they did us, and we were capturing guns and ammunition galore. We kept them on the run until we got to the Marne, where they turned around to make a fight. just what we wanted. This was, I think, the tenth or eleventh of September. The battle lasted two days and we didn't half give them something. We popped them off as fast as the clock could tick at times. At last they were forced to retire. As fast as they retired we followed them up until night came, and we had a good night's rest without being disturbed.

We started next morning straight into action. My regiment got some hand to hand fighting this day in a village. We got in close quarters with the bayonet and we let them feel it. We captured the village and many prisoners and also left a few hundred dead there. Then we came to the Aisne. Here they held us in check a few hours until word came that we must cross the bridge today at all costs. We did, but not without great loss. This was at midday on the thirteenth of September. The remainder of that day there was heavy cannonading on both sides, but we held our position, which had cost us dearly.

We were now in Soissons. That night my regiment was on outpost duty and it was pouring heavens hard with rain and we laid out in the open. We were like drowned rats next morning when we got relieved, but we got a nice day's rest, for we had got a good position. We were in a long deep nullah out of sight from the enemy and it was only about twelve feet wide. They would have to be very accurate if they wanted to drop a shell in it. The Germans were shelling us very heavy all that day and our side hardly ever fired a round, only now and again the artillery would fire one.. We wondered what the matter was, but we found out later we were short of ammunition. That is why we could not advance any further.

The enemy's shells were flying over our heads and dropping short all that day, but they could not hit our mark. We got so used to them we took no notice of them at the finish. Night time came and the shelling ceased, but as soon as daybreak came the shelling started again. Still we took no notice, until about midday an enemy aeroplane hovered over us for about half an hour and then returned to his own line, and soon a shell dropped straight into the nullah. I got it along with five others wounded and one killed. One of the wounded was my captain. I lay there only about ten minutes, then I was picked up by our stretcher bearers and carried to an old church about a quarter of a mile away. There I saw my captain. He was laid next to me. We got our wounds attended to and stayed there until midnight, and all the time we were there the enemy were shelling the church. Luckily we got away without further injury. They dared not move us in the day time because we had to cross the bridge again, and the enemy had the range on it. We were moved at midnight and went away in ambulance wagons to another dressing station, then, after being dressed, we left there at once in motor wagons and arrived at another dressing station, where our wounds were dressed again and we were taken to the railway station. We were placed in cattle trucks and then we started on our journey. We traveled all night and until noon the next day. Then they took us from the cattle trucks and placed us on a railway platform, and it was to my delight for I never experienced such a ride in my life. I expected to arrive at Paris in pieces. They gave us a good feed, then the doctor came round and picked out the worst cases and told us we were to be taken to the American Ambulance, which was about ten miles from the station.

We were placed in ambulance cars at once. Here again I saw my captain. He was put in the same car as myself, and we had a good chat together. We arrived at the hospital about 4 p. m. I was taken to a nice clean bed, bathed and made as comfortable as possible, and I am sure there is not a hospital anywhere where a wounded man could get better attended to.

CHAPTER V.

THE AMERICAN AMBULANCE OF JUILLY.

What a change to be transferred from the great bustling city of Paris to this quiet little village of Juilly! Although but 23 miles distant from Paris, yet it took us two hours to make the trip from the Gare du Nord to the tiny station of St. Mard. Numerous troop trains having the right of way delayed the passenger traffic, as they do all over that part of France where there is military activity. American workers at Neuilly, in France for the first time in their lives, have difficulty in making fellow-mortals understand their pronunciation of the word Neuilly. The word Juilly exacts an equal number of variations in pronunciation. Perhaps there are no two names in French geography harder to pronounce correctly and, curiously enough, these two places were chosen for the two hospitals of the American Ambulance. One of our doctors who had just arrived from America took the wrong trains in Paris and found himself at Meaux. It was a rainy night, he was carrying a heavy suit-case and he did not know a word of French. He wandered around trying to find someone who could understand his pronunciation of Juilly. After trying without success every combination of sound that he could think of he was about to conclude that the place did not exist, when he thought of writing the name on a piece of paper.

When Mrs. H. P. Whitney, in December, 1914, offered to equip and maintain a hospital for French wounded soldiers, several locations were offered by the government and the college of Juilly was finally chosen. The institution lies between two main railways running toward the battle line, and at that time was considered quite near the front. If you look at a map of France you will not in all probability find Juilly, as it is a village of only some 400 inhabitants. The name Juilly is derived from Julius, and it is thought that at one time Julius Caesar had a camp there. At any rate, we know that the Romans invaded this part of Gaul and in the College Park is a splendid Roman wine jar which has been unearthed and mounted on a pedestal at the end of an avenue of elm trees.

The College was founded in 1630 by the Oratorians and was made a royal academy by Louis XIII. Some famous men have been students here, as Villars, d'Artagnan, Montesquieu, Norfolk, Howard d'Arundel and Jérôme Napoleon. The great Napoleon came here once to see his brother Jérôme and the room where he slept is pointed out to visitors, also a framed letter on the wall in which Napoleon gives his brother good advice as to his school behavior.

It was not a new experience for the College to receive wounded soldiers, for it was used as a hospital both in the wars of the French revolution and in the Franco-Prussian war. At the battle of the Marne 500 wounded were brought here and covered the floors of the corridors, and German prisoners were locked up in a room which was afterwards used as our kitchen.

The buildings are a sturdy pile of three storied stone structures with little pretense to architectural merit. Only the northeast wing and the college theatre are used for the wounded with accommodations for 220. The rest of the college is intact and instruction of the youth of France continues as in the times of peace. One of the charming features of the place is the park in the rear of the buildings. Here are wide lawns, beautiful avenues of elm trees and a small lake, the home of snow-white swans.

The Americans early in 1915 had a busy time of it converting the old stone building with walls four feet or more in thickness and devoid of all plumbing, into a building of modern hospital requirements. Workmen were mobilized with the army, and it was with the greatest difficulty that men could be obtained to install the plumbing, heating and electric lighting systems. All the material had to be assembled in Paris and hauled out in trucks, some of the hauls requiring two days. The spring of St. Geneviève was tapped and water pumped to cisterns on the roof. Electricity was brought from a one-horse concern at the village of St. Mard , about two miles away. A central heating plant and sewer system were installed and the necessary equipment of an up-to-date hospital completed.

The little village is a quaint affair as are most French villages. There is the town square lined with linden trees in front of the college and across the square is the village church. There is of course the Mairie and l'École des Garçons et l'École des Filles. The mayor is a well preserved man of sturdy stock whose only son is in the trenches. The mayor's wife is a sweet, admirable woman living in constant dread of hearing bad news about her son. Yet she would not have him back in safety, as she knows he is fighting for France and for her loved ones. We, in America, have too little thought of the noble French women who are on their knees every day praying that the bitter cup may pass them by, but meeting their sorrow with wonderful resignation if this prayer is denied them.

There are a few stores selling general merchandise, the butcher shop, the pork shop (always a separate institution in France), little fruit, tobacco and newspaper shops and several estaminets or wine shops. The post office and telephone are directed by two or three intelligent women. Mail is delivered from Juilly to surrounding hamlets and is carried by a young widow. In good weather she rides a bicycle, but in bad weather she does her ten miles a day on foot. Her husband was killed in the battle of the Marne, leaving her with a young child, alone and unprovided. "Yes," she says, "life is hard. I am left a widow with a young child, but my husband died for France and that means that he died defending me and my son and the other women and children of France." She never complains as she trudges along the muddy roads in the rain, and she always has a cheerful smile for the Americans.

There are two shoemakers, the tile-roof man and the village carpenter and blacksmith. The last two are expert artisans and are of great service to the Ambulance. Of inns there are none at all. The village is too small to support one. Likewise with the gendarmes. There is an antiquated garde champêtre who fixes official notices on the Mairie and at times goes through the streets ringing a bell and reading governmental announcements.

The hospital is glad to get village help for the laundry and kitchen but with so much work to be done in their homes it is difficult to get women workers. However, there are over fifty women from Juilly and surrounding villages who work in the laundry and kitchen, and act as ward maids and scrub women.

The staff consists of a varying number of doctors, most of them Americans, twenty to twenty-five trained nurses, several auxiliary nurses and some volunteer orderlies. There is an automobile ambulance section attached to the hospital. Most of the drivers are young men from the United States and they drive Ford cars which are fitted to carry three lying-down patients or couchés.

For some months the wounded were received from Compiègne, which is about seven miles from the trenches. This made a run of about thirty miles in ambulances which was too severe for badly wounded men, especially in bad weather. Besides that, the possibility of the hospital being kept full of patients depended on the activity of that

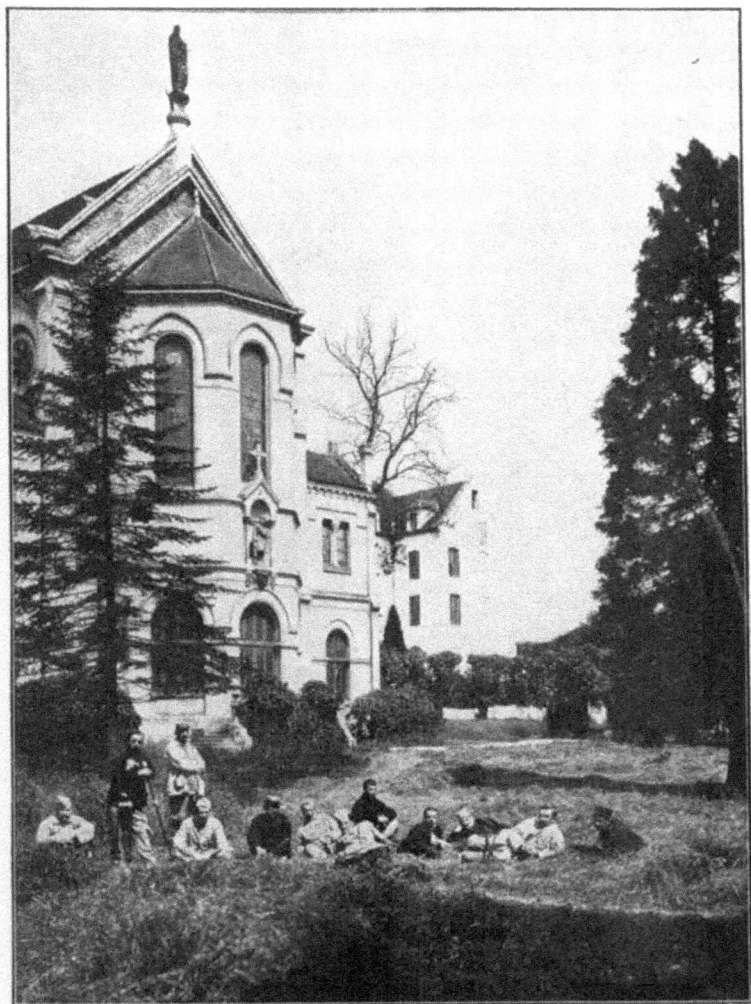

The American Ambulance branch hospital in the College of Juilly.

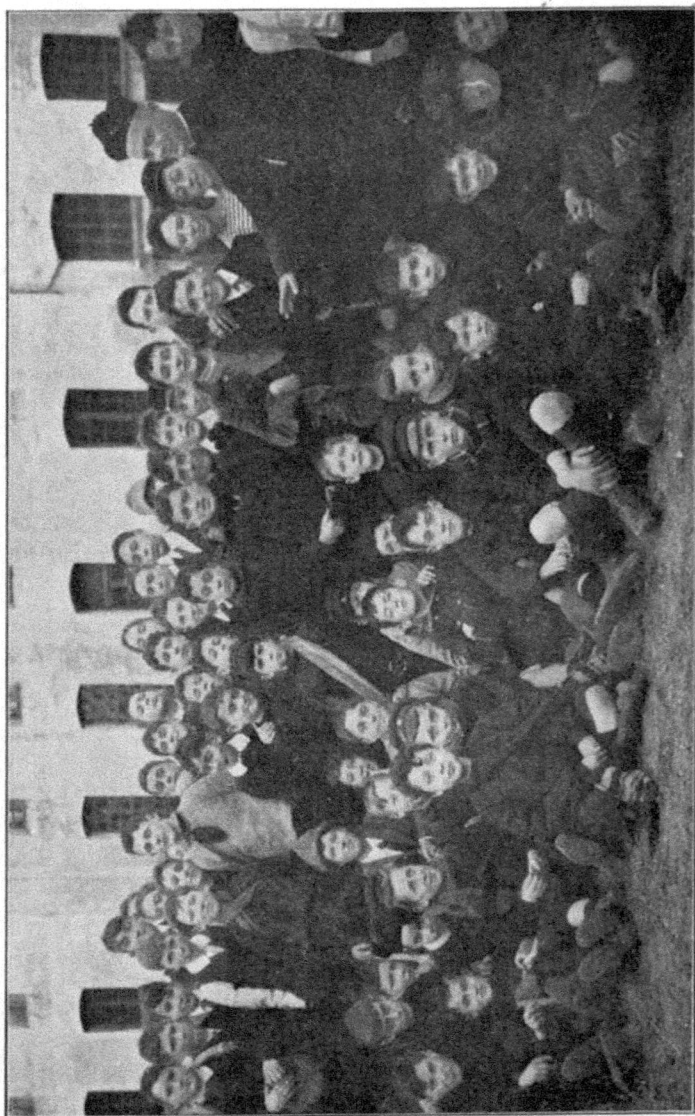

School boys of the College of Juilly

section of the line and when there were few or no engagements there were no wounded to be had. Later on a different arrangement was made whereby the hospital, although geographically in the Zone des Armées, was included in the Camp Retranché de Paris. This system was much more advantageous, as wounded were received from along the battle line from Verdun to the Somme.

The guns at the front can be heard every day at Juilly. Our first great sensation in the war zone was an indescribable thrill when we heard the cannon booming in the distance towards Soissons. The sound, now louder now fainter, when heard for the first time cannot fail to make an impression. This voice of death blown by the winds over the fields and ruined villages of France brings a consciousness of the reality of war as does no other sound. To one who has not heard it, the sensation cannot be imparted. To one who has heard it, the memory will never be forgotten.

CHAPTER VI.

LIFE IN THE AMBULANCE.

We find at once a great difference between the living here and at Neuilly. At Neuilly, while of course the patients were French, yet it was essentially an American hospital and English was spoken freely. Here we live in much more intimacy with the French and a speaking knowledge of the language is essential if one wants to be of the greatest service. Accordingly we looked around for a teacher and found that the housekeeper's daughter gave lessons. She was a buxom French girl of 19 with a perfect American accent.

"Where did you learn to speak English so well?" we asked her.

"Oh, I went to school in America for eight months."

"In what part of America were you?"

"I was in Honolulu at the Punahou School."

Then she told us how her parents had taken her some years before to Australia and not wanting to stay there decided to return to France by way of America. They had stopped off at Honolulu, where she had gone to school and although since then she had not had much opportunity to practise speaking English she had never forgotten what she had learned.

Our bedroom is across the hall from one of the large wards and was formerly one of the professor's rooms. It is convenient to be so near the blessés, as when one is called at night for a hemorrhage, it doesn't take long to get there.

The daily routine is as follows. Breakfast of café au lait, toast and eggs at 7 a. m. We drink our coffee out of bowls to save crockery and eat off an oil cloth covered table to save laundry. "Rounds" at 9 a. m. After which dressings are done. The poilus have their lunch at eleven and the staff at noon. The déjeuner is the best meal of the day and consists of some kind of meat or fish, two or three vegetables, sometimes a salad and cheese and coffee. We are in the Brie region and a ripe Brie cheese is delicious.

If there are operations to be done, these commence at 1:30 p. m. The operating room is well equipped and the technique is excellent. In the afternoon we usually take a walk and roam around the surrounding country. There is a tennis court located in a grove of elm trees in the park where we play occasionally. It seems strange to play tennis while we can hear cannon booming in the distance and aeroplanes occasionally sail over our heads.

Supper is served at 7 p. m., and is a plain meal of meat, vegetables and fruit. In the evenings we read or indulge in a game of ping-pong in one of the long stone corridors.

Among our blessés are a number of Algerians. They are fine looking fellows with well-shaped heads. They seem quiet and docile, but on dit that they are demons in a fight. They do not like the cold weather and the trench warfare. Under their quiet demeanor is a quick temper. One day when a band of a passing regiment was giving a concert in the courtyard and the soldiers were crowded around the musicians, we heard a loud crack of something breaking and discovered that an Algerian in a fit of sudden rage had broken his cane over a French soldier's head and knocked him senseless. There was nothing to do but carry the soldier on a stretcher to his bed and "evacuate" the offender at once to his dépôt. The Arabs do not know what to make of having women nurses around. They call them "Mees" or "Mama" and the stout nurses are greatly in favor. They want to take the fat ones back to Algeria with them.

Two of our cars go three times a week to Compiègne for wounded and it is a fine ride. Our route passes through Dammartin, finely situated on a hill, where General French had his headquarters at one time. We then follow along a smooth road passing through several picturesque villages to the beautiful forest of Ermenonville. In Dumas "Three Musketeers," he speaks of his heroes riding from Dammartin to Ermenonville in ten minutes. Perhaps horses went faster in those heroic days, for it takes us fully twenty minutes in a Ford. On strategic points everywhere are barbed wire entanglements and here and there are cleverly constructed reserve trenches. The French are taking no chances and if the Germans ever break through they will not find it easy going. There has been no hunting allowed since the war started and the game is very tame. Fat pheasants and partridges scurry across the road, occasionally we see a hare or a herd of deer and the lake at Ermenonville is dotted with wild ducks. The ancient village of Verberie is passed through on the way. Here the English king Ethelwolf was married to Judith over a thousand years ago. Shortly afterwards, where the railway crosses the road, sentries stop the cars and our papers are carefully examined before we are allowed to proceed. The forest of Compiegne is magnificent and it is not strange that it was a favorite resort of the French royalty. The handsome town of Compiègne seems very peaceful considering it is seven miles or so from the trenches. Some of the residences are closed but most of the stores are open, people were sitting on the sidewalk cafés and carriages were driving through the streets. The large château of Louis XV, where Napoleon met his bride Marie Louise, is now used as a receiving hospital, and thither we repair for our allotment of wounded.

One day a Taube dropped a bomb on the courtyard about twenty minutes before our arrival, and a large hole occupied the place where we usually stationed our cars. The bomb broke most of the windows of the palace, peppered the walls and wounded a few hospital attendants. The statues in the hallways of the château are padded with straw and boxed up as a protection, but if a bomb should make a square hit, it didn't seem as if such measures would be of much avail. Usually there is some waiting for the wounded to arrive, so we have time to see something of the park with its splendid vistas, the handsome Hôtel de Ville and the statue of Joan of Arc. It was here that Joan was captured. How much of the spirit of that heroic maid is breathed in France today!

A visit to Dr. Carrel's hospital is a rare treat. The hospital is established in a fine hotel and it is an ideal institution, although an occasional shell which drops in the garden makes the proximity to the trenches not an unmixed blessing. Dr. Carrel was conducting his researches on the treatment of wounds which later became known as the "Carrel-Dakin method," and is a notable achievement in war surgery.

The sound of the cannon is very loud at Compiègne and other evidences of the proximity of the enemy are the destroyed bridge over the Oise, and several residences in the town utterly ruined by shell fire.

When the wounded come in and our quota is received we hurry back to Juilly. We wrap the blessés well in blankets and have hot coffee in thermos bottles for use en route. Where the road is rough, care is taken to jolt the wounded as little as possible. On arriving at the ambulance the wounded are undressed. They are nearly always very dirty and very tired. Their uniforms are caked with dirt and blood. They are given a hot bath if they are able to have it. Joly, the Major Domo of the receiving room, is quite a character. As soon as a wounded man is turned over to him he seats him on a slat arrangement which lies across the tub. Then with a bottle of liquid soap and a sponge he goes at his job with zest. First a thorough shampoo, Joly keeping up a running fire of conversation, and if the soap runs down the victim's face and into his eyes and mouth, Joly doesn't mind it a bit but follows up with liberal douches of hot water. The poilu seems to enjoy it all as much as Joly. A soldier, badly wounded or with fracture of the leg, is carefully bathed on a bed, and is not subject to Joly's ministrations. All the wounded are X-rayed unless it is very evident that the wound is merely a flesh wound. Cases requiring immediate operation are attended to at once. Sometimes the electric light system breaks down at the critical moment and acetylene lamps are ready for emergencies. The poor fellows are put to bed and given a meal and the inevitable cigarette. They then sleep and sleep. Many of them have not been in a bed for months. They usually sleep all night, all the next day, waking up only for meals, the next night and part of the next day. Quite often they have bad dreams and nightmares and cry out in their sleep as they dream of an attack.

CHAPTER VII.

THE SURROUNDING COUNTRY.

On the road to Paris, about a mile and a half away, is the village of Nantouillet, which is distinguished by a fine old château built by Charles de Melun, grand master of France under Louis XI. The moat and ivy covered walls are still well preserved and the building shows some charming architectural features. The present master of the Château is a prisoner in Germany and his efficient wife manages the farm. Before the battle of the Marne a squad of Uhlans rode into her courtyard and selected the best dog out of a famous kennel of hunting dogs. The Germans seemed to have been well informed about France even to small details. This reminds me of the story of the professor in the college.

For some time before the war began there had been a German on the faculty at Juilly. It was noticed that he spent most of his time outside of class work in walks and bicycle rides around the country. A few days before war was declared he disappeared. On the battlefield of the Marne, a few weeks later, his dead body was found clad in a German officer's uniform. In his pockets were well-drawn maps of the surrounding country, showing every road, hill, wood and stream of military value.

A few miles away is the pleasing château of St. Thibault on a large estate. The charming and cultivated family were fond of Americans and entertained us during the summer months.

The neighboring village of Thieux is notable for its attractive little church which was visited, according to the records, by Joan of Arc on August 13, 1429.

The Seine et Marne is one of the most fertile parts of France. The country is mostly flat, with low lying hills, clumps of woods, meadows and fields. There is no waste land. Toward the east are great stretches of wheat fields. A year ago these fields were red with blood, but nature rapidly effaces the signs of war and wheat is now waving over the fields destined to rank in history with Châlons and Tours.

Perched on a hill and a land mark from our hospital windows is the town of Montgé. Some British troops came through here in the retreat from Mons and blew up two houses in order to barricade the street, but the Germans came along on the other side of the hill. Now there is an artillery force stationed here. On our first visit the woods on the hill were full of soldiers digging trenches and we saw two of the fatuous "seventy-fives." They were painted over to resemble leaves, also a wire netting was spread over them which can be covered with branches and conceal the cannon from hostile aviators.

Along the road to Meaux is the newly-made cemetery where 317 soldiers are buried, among them Péguy, the young poet whom France mourns. These men were killed the night before the 6th of September, 1914, when Joffre gave his famous order that they should retreat no further, and that they should die in their tracks rather than give way. A body of troops was bivouacking in the field and a German battery on the hill of Monthyon got their range and landed several shell in their midst. The graves are decorated with metallic wreaths, and among them is one from the American Ambulance. Nearby is a plot where Germans are buried. It is fenced off with barbed wire and a black post with a board and number marks the spot. How magnanimous of the French to protect and care for the graves of the ruthless invaders of their country!

Meaux is the nearest large town to us and is probably the largest town nearest to Paris that the Germans reached in 1914. A good part of the population fled on the approach of the enemy. Only German patrols entered the town. The main bodies of troops never had a chance as they were engaged in heavy fighting on the outskirts by the French.

Dr. Gros of the American Ambulance tells a vivid story which shows what the French soldier endured in these glorious days of the Marne. With other Americans from Paris, Dr. Gros went out to the battlefield to bring in the wounded. They arrived at Meaux at midnight and found the town in darkness. There was not a light to be seen or a sound to be heard except the wailings of cats, wandering around the streets. They called and shouted and at last were able to arouse an official. "Where are the wounded?" they asked. "I will show you," replied the official. They were led with the aid of a lamp to a school building which looked dark and deserted. Pushing open the door they found the building crowded with wounded, over five hundred. They were lying on the hard floor. Some were dead, others dying, all were asleep. Nine days of forced marching and fighting without adequate sleep or food had produced such a state of exhaustion that they wanted only to be left alone. The prospect of surgical care, hospital, food and drink aroused no response. The worst cases were selected first, such as compound fractures and those wounded in the chest or abdomen. They made little or no complaint when they were picked up. Only when their wounds, stuck to the floor, were torn open, did they utter a sound.

Further along up the beautiful Marne valley, about an hour's ride from Meaux, lies the attractive town of Château Thierry, of about 7,000 inhabitants. Here La Fontaine, the fable writer, was born. The castle that gives the town its name is a 1200-year old ruin, picturesquely situated on the high bank of the Marne.

German troops crossed the river here in their great advance but were driven back again after the battle of the Marne, blowing up the bridge as they retreated, and British and French troops made the crossing on pontoons. The town suffered somewhat from shell fire and numerous shell holes are to be seen as grim reminders of the war. Because Château Thierry is located deep in the valley the sound of the guns at the front is not heard and there is little to make one realize that war is going on.

In company with some French officers I visited the hospitals and lunched at the officers' mess. Questions about America and the American ambulance from a score of officers I answered as best I could and they were too polite to notice my mistakes in the French language. The Médecin-Chef of the hospitals was a very nervous man, drafted from civil life and breaking under the strain of his office. When I said "merci" in refusing a dish offered me, he thundered at me "Merci oui ou merci non?" which amused everybody.

In a large enclosure in the town were a number of freshly captured, unwounded German prisoners. The officers were very sour and surly-looking. The privates were youths with closely cropped heads and seemed not at all sorry to be prisoners. They were kindly treated by the French and received the same food as the French soldiers.

CHAPTER VIII.

THE WOUNDED FROM THE BATTLE OF CHAMPAGNE.

During the fall of 1915 there were rumors of a great offensive to be made somewhere along the line. Although we were within sound of the guns we knew little of what was going on and often read in New York papers of events that was news to us, days old. Early in September we received orders to evacuate all of our blessés who were able to go. Then there was a great scurry, filling out the military papers, getting out the equipment and bidding farewell to the poilus who had been so long with us and to whom we had grown so attached. We waited expectantly every day for news of a great battle until on September 26th the official communiqués announced that, preceded by a heavy bombardment, the French had advanced in the Champagne region and had taken many prisoners and trenches. We were prepared to receive a load of wounded at any time.

September 29th we were notified by telegram that a trainload of wounded would arrive at five o'clock the next morning, and we were ready when the ambulances began to arrive from the station of St. Mard in rapid succession, each one with three wounded. One man died at the station before he could be taken off the train. The long corridor was filled with wounded, wrapped in blankets lying on stretchers, and as rapidly as possible the blessés were carried up to the wards, the worst cases first. In less than three hours from the arrival of the first patient the last of the 128 was put to bed. Extra cars and drivers had been sent out from Neuilly else we never could have handled the task so rapidly.

A large man lay in the corridor, his head so swathed in bandages that all of his face that could be seen was a nose, a pair of large moustaches and a pair of keen gray eyes. I picked up the head end of the stretcher and our Belgian radiographer, Deschamps, the foot end and we carried him up two flights of stairs. He grew heavier and heavier until, as we reached the bed our aching arms had some difficulty in raising the stretcher sufficiently to make the transfer to the bed. As we were struggling with our task we were startled to hear a voice roar at us out of the maze of bandages and blankets, "Brace up there! Brace up." Our patient turned out to be a colonel who spoke perfect English, a magnificent specimen, 6 feet 4 and 245 pounds weight. As soon as we learned his rank we hurried and prepared a private room for him.

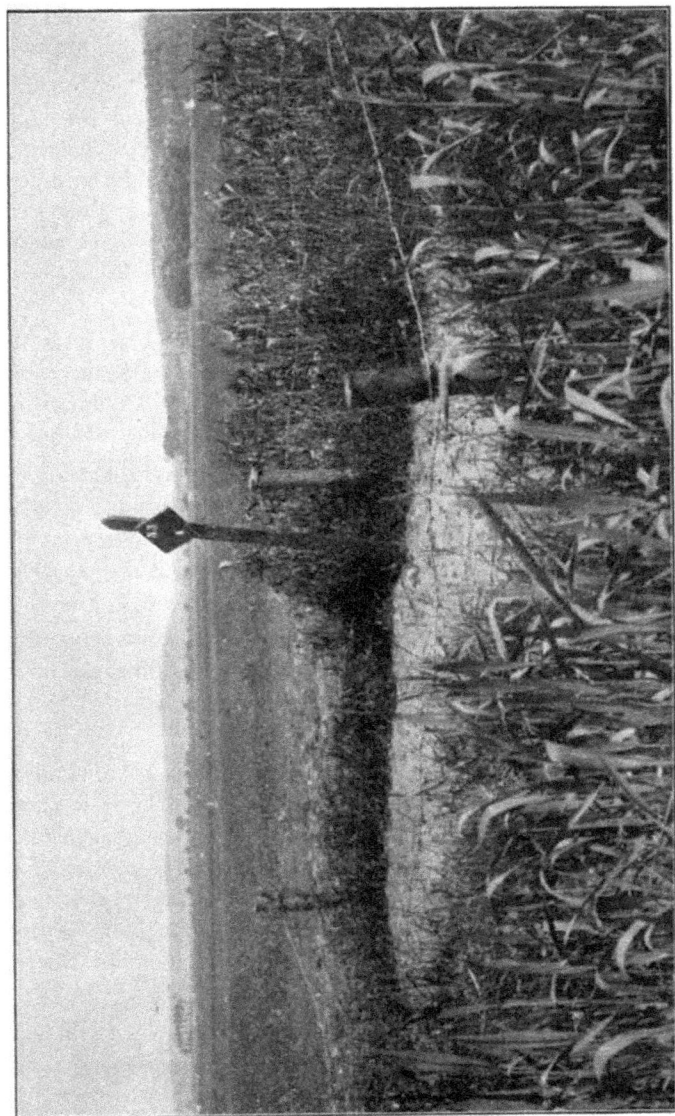

A cemetery of German dead on the battlefield of the Marne, cared for by the French government.

Every patient was then examined and dressed. Some were in desperate condition and had to be operated on at once. There were some terrible wounds, especially the jaw cases. It does not seem possible that a man could be alive with such wounds. One boy was shot through the shoulder at close range, then the ball tore open his neck and carried away a good part of the lower jaw, floor of the mouth and tongue. He was a nervous little chap and suffered greatly. He was fed by a tube introduced into his nose, but did not look as if he could survive.

Another, boy was shot through the face sideways, the piece of shell tearing away a large part of the lower jaw and half his tongue. A fringe of lower lip hung down almost to his chest. He cannot speak, so writes notes asking for something to drink and whether he will ever be able to speak again. He is wonderfully brave and patient and after having been fed a few times he took his tube, funnel and pitcher of milk and insisted on feeding himself.

One fine young fellow has his leg shattered and gas gangrene has set in. It is too late to save him. His mother arrives from Paris. He sees her entering the door, cries out "Mama" and holds out his hands to her. She rushes to him and folds him in her arms-her only son. He expires before long but with a peaceful smile on his face.

We are busy as can be, for as fast as a round of dressings is completed we must start again, as they are so quickly soiled. When we get a chance to think it over, anger takes possession of us—rage that boys and young men, the flower of the land, should thus be struck down and mutilated in defending their country and dear ones from the merciless greed of the Kaiser and his cohorts.

The stench in the ward is beyond description. One of our old patients is helping with the dressings, and although he has been wounded four times and has gone back again to the trenches, the smell is too much for him and he vomits repeatedly but always returns to help.

The saddest cases of all are the blind. Dr. Scarlett comes out from Paris to do what he can for them, but too often their eyesight has gone beyond hope. It is heart-rending to witness their hope when they recover from the anaesthetic and believe, now that they have been attended to by the American doctor, they will be all right. They get some one to light a cigarette for them, laugh and crack jokes. Later on when the consciousness that they are doomed to everlasting darkness comes to them, they are magnificent. Not a whimper, a word of sorrow or self-pity passes their lips. They meet their fate with the noble fortitude of the race.

The nurses are working splendidly and are at their best now that there is plenty of work. The first night was a terrible one, but we managed to get through it with a liberal use of morphine. Almost every patient is bad enough to require a special nurse in civil practice, and for our 52 patients in a ward we have three nurses and one auxiliary. There are no trained orderlies, but the convalescent soldiers rapidly become apt helpers. If war brutalizes soldiers, it certainly does not show itself in the attitude of the French soldiers to each other, as no one could be more solicitous and tender than are these poilus of their fellow comrades.

And so it goes on. A few die, those who were hopeless on their arrival. The village priest is called and gives them the last rites. Gradually conditions improve, the blessés suffer less and the stench in the wards diminishes. But just as we feel relieved that no more of our blessés are going to die, the danger of secondary hemorrhages arises. These come on suddenly and without warning, as the infection reaches and ulcerates an artery. One night I was called to the ward hurriedly and by the light of a lantern was appalled to see blood pouring out of a man's mouth. The poor fellow was choking and blood poured all over the bed. There was no success in trying to see where the blood came from. A shrapnel ball had struck him in the face alongside of the nose and traversed the neck and the blood poured out of his mouth too fast to sponge it out and see by lantern light the source of the bleeding. A finger in his mouth felt a hole in his hard palate through which the blood poured and the finger was used to plug the hole until the blood could be cleaned out and the wound packed. By this time the blessé was white as a sheet, sitting up in bed covered with blood. Two tears rolled down his cheeks as he said "Merci," kissed my hand and settled back on his pillows.

This afternoon as I was shaving an Algerian who had his upper jaw smashed by a bullet, I heard a splashing sound and an old chap came staggering into the salle de pansements with blood pouring out from a great hole in his face. He started to bleed as he sat up in bed and, knowing that I was in the dressing room, he came in there after me, leaving a trail of blood behind him. Vigorous packing stopped the hemorrhage for the time being but later on it was necessary to tie the external carotid artery in his neck. We call this poilu "grandpère," for, although he is only thirty-nine, yet he has only a fringe of gray locks around the edge of his bald pate A Chinese bullet fifteen years ago carried away a part of his nose and a piece of German shell took away most of what was left and a large piece of his upper jaw. When he was wounded, grandpère crawled into a shell hole and packed his wound full of mud to stop the bleeding. He is a Breton fisherman and makes long fishing voyages to the Canadian banks. He knows two English words, "Cod fish" and "Whisky."

After a varying length of time in the hospital the blessés are evacuated. The slightly wounded ones go to their dépôt, where they receive permission to visit their families for a few weeks before their return to the trenches. Those requiring further treatment are sent to convalescent hospitals in Paris or its suburbs. The hopelessly crippled men go before a Board and are reforméd, that is, the war is over for them. They go home and do what they can to make a living. Partially disabled soldiers are placed in the auxiliary service, where they are assigned to work in accordance with their capacity as drivers, railroad helpers, kitchen assistants, hospital orderlies or workers in ammunition factories.

Some of our wounded speak English quite well. A bright young fellow from Soissons who had never been a hundred miles away from home spoke English and was glad of the opportunity to improve his knowledge of the language. He had learned English in the college at Soissons and the result was a striking improvement over the success of an American boy learning French at an American college. At our request he wrote out a story of his experiences in the war, the first part in French and the "most interesting part of the story" in English.

CHAPTER IX.

ROBERT'S STORY.

I was at my home north of Soissons when the war broke out. I was nineteen years of age and I did not expect at that time that I would be called to the colors.

The first of September, 1914, French troops retreating from Charleroi had just passed through our village when cries of terror resounded in the streets, "Les Allemands, les Uhlans." We heard in the distance the clatter of horses' hoofs and some minutes later the Belgian lancers, then the artillery passed at full speed. It was a false alarm. The "Boches" were our friends, the Belgians.

After this my mother, who did not want me to remain in the village during the invasion, made preparations for my departure. In the evening as we learned from the dragoons, the last troops in retreat, that the Germans were only 12 kilometers away, I bade my parents farewell and started on foot for Paris. All night long I walked. It was a terrible night for me. Behind me the cannon thundered over our poor villages and the glare of flaming homes, burned by the enemy, added a note of horror to this first vision of war. I trudged all night long with death in my soul, 43 kilometres, thinking of my family in the hands of the enemy. I began to understand what war was. A year later I had to understand it more.

I was ordered to report to a regiment at Paris, and then was sent to a camp for instruction. Sickness delayed my departure for the front so that it was not until June that I joined my comrades in the trenches of the Aisne. Our regiment held a secteur violently bombarded day and night, only a few kilometres from my home town.

By the middle of August we were ordered to the Champagne region to prepare for the approaching offensive. There we dug by night new trenches and "boyaux." Our lines, 800 meters distant from the enemy, were moved up to 400 and even 300 metres. During the day we dug our old "boyaux" deeper.

On September 20th we learned the decision of the Commander in Chief. We were going to take the offensive in a few days. When our turn came for guard duty in the first line we sewed the traditional square of white cloth on our knapsacks, which would denote our presence to our artillery and prevent our being shot by our own men.

The twenty-second of September at five o'clock in the morning we took our place in the first line. Two sections of my company were on guard and the two others were at rest in the dug-outs. As for myself I fell asleep at once in a dug-out as I was very tired. Suddenly about seven o'clock an infernal noise awoke me all of a sudden. The "seventy-fives" near us fired all at once and in about an hour all of our "seventy-fives" were engaged. The Boches replied. The "seventy-sevens," "one hundred and fives" and "one hundred and fifties" were rained on our batteries but without effect.

A sergeant entered our dug-out all excited, "Here is the order," he said. "The offensive has started, the bombardment will last three or four days. The seventy-fives

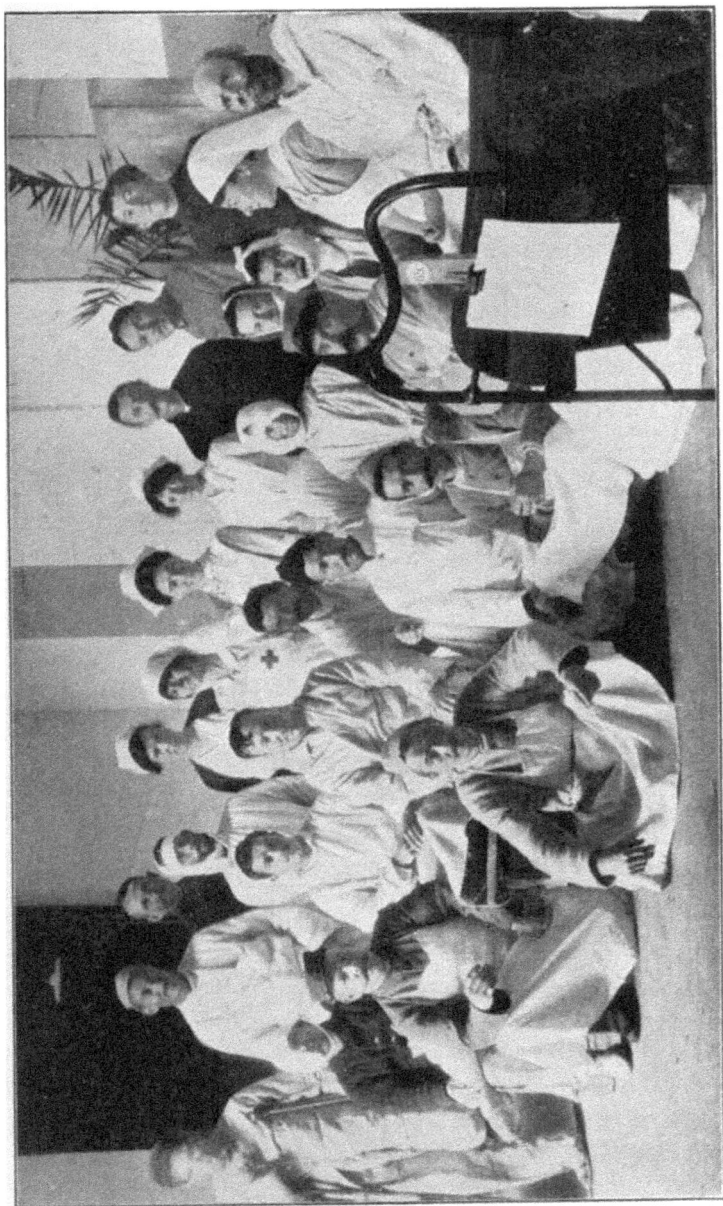

Dr. and Mrs. Judd with a group of poilus and nurses at Juilly

will fire today, tomorrow the heavy cannon and on the last day all the artillery will fire at the same time. At the attack you will be the first to go." His words are received without a murmur. We then crack jokes as the Boche shells continue to fall above us causing some caving in of the ceilings of our dug-outs. At last towards midday the Boche quit firing. As for us, our bombardment became more and more intense.

The third day of the bombardment must have been a terrible one for the enemy. Shells of all sizes threw up into the air for hundreds of feet pieces of rocks, trees and material of various kinds. The explosions of our "75" and "155" and of our aerial torpedoes on the enemy's first lines confused our brains and upset our stomachs.

The twenty-fourth of September we learned that on the next day at nine fifteen exactly our company would be the first to attack and take the first line of the enemy's trenches. The news hardly surprised us as we expected it. Some of us were chosen as "trench cleaners" or "zigouilleurs" and received a strong knife and a Browning revolver. The "trench cleaner's" duty is during an attack to kill all the enemy hidden in the dug-outs who would be able to shoot us in the back.

During the night we prepared our sacks, containing three days of reserve rations and saw to our square of white cloth which would guide our artillery.

Here I speak English for the most interesting part of the story.

Twenty-fifth of September. It is eight o'clock in the morning. We are ready. With our sack we have also two musettes; one for grenades and cartridges, and the other for chocolate and bread. To our belts are hung a set of small tools and a "pochette", holding the masque and pad designed to ward off the asphyxiating gases. Last, we each have two "bidons" of a capacity of one litre apiece.

For myself I also carry a board two meters long which I am to lay across the foremost enemy trench to allow the passage of my comrades. In the right hand, my rifle.

It rains, and this depresses us a little; but we are accustomed by former duties to all the caprices of the weather and rain is not going to hinder our determination.

Our lieutenant calls the section together. He tells us that we shall be the first to move; we are to be the regiment's first wave of assault. We are told to leap over the parapet at fifteen minutes past nine and to then march straight before us in the direction of Sommepy-Vouziers, in short, towards the north. "I know," says our lieutenant, "that there is not one of you who will show any sign of weakness." Our glance suffices to convince him that, every one, we are proud to attack first, and that, among us, none shall recoil. "Tomorrow morning," continues our lieutenant, "we shall have forced the lines of the enemy. We shall be at Sommepy. It will be Sunday and we shall attend high mass which will be celebrated by soldier priests in the ruins of the church." Saluting, we return to our arms.

The rain falls, drizzling yet heavy. The bombardment becomes more and more violent, the bursting of our terrible 75s falling from far before us, often into our own trenches, bringing danger to us from our own comrades. We feel a great enthusiasm course through us more and more; among us there is not one who glances back with regret upon other days in this hour of death. Each gazes, on the contrary, frankly

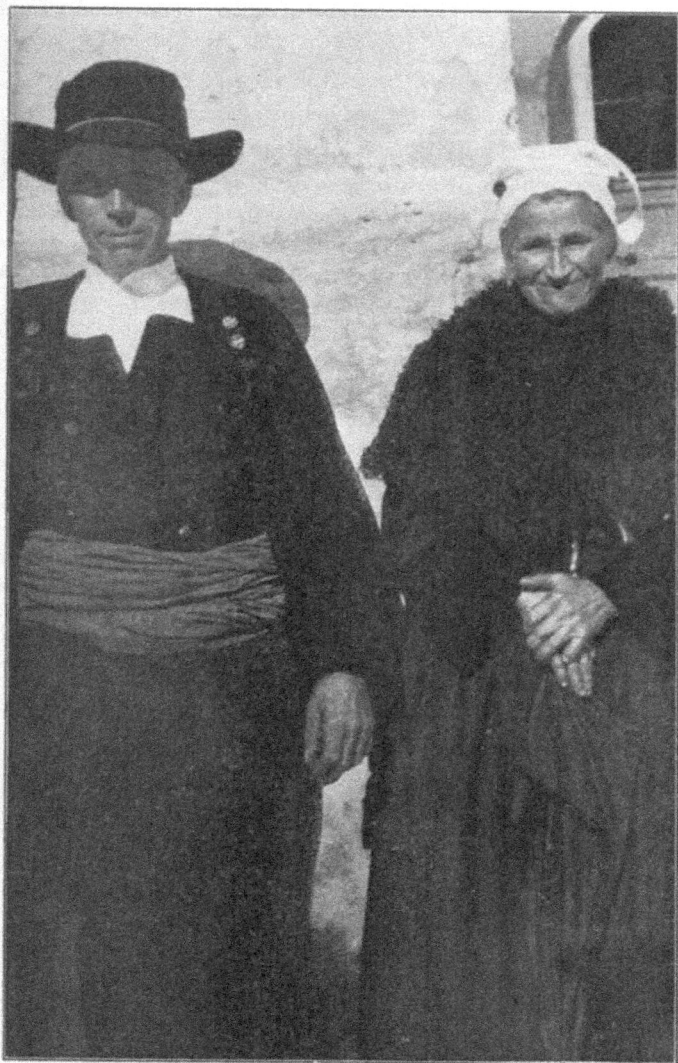

Breton Peasants who have come to visit their son who is badly wounded.

towards that future which looms up as red as the blood which is soon going to dye that "plateau." Everyone thinks "our life would have been worth something for would we not have aided in saving our France from danger?" We smoke a pipe; we speak of the terrible moments that we are about to live and which we foresee as less terrible than the reality.

At last! nine o'clock has come. The section files into the "parallèle," a trench with steps dug during the night before our first line to aid the movements of the appointed hour.

"Du courage, mes enfants," cries our lieutenant; "regret nothing; think of that future which is dawning so beautifully for France, that future which will be your glory and your recompense. Not one of you will retreat. The moment has come for us to drive the invader from our land and to restore those innumerable ruined places which you will see on your way. Remember that you are soldiers of the glorious Thirty-fifth Infantry Regiment of Belfort."

The lieutenant lights his pipe; we put bayonet to rifle, musette to back and adjust our helmets.

Five minutes past nine * * * the artillery is increasing its range. The attack is going to begin. How very long seem these moments.

Ten minutes past nine * * * Ready, mes enfants, to the escaliers! We embrace; fathers gaze for a last moment upon photographs of wives and children, confide to them their last thoughts as they press kisses upon them. * * * Unforgetable minutes, of which still the memory horrifies yet fascinates me. Once more I see a fine, heavy-bearded comrade of the "Bresse" embracing his sergeant as bearded as himself while he mutters, "An revoir, et non adieu." This scene is chiselled into my memory.

Fifteen minutes past nine! Our lieutenant climbs the parapet of the trench and, raising his sword: "En avant mes enfants, and good luck!"

From this moment, cruel minutes passed through my mind for not having full consciousness of the reality, I lived as in a dream, asking myself always if in this hour men were surely about to spill each other's blood. Here is best what I remember:

My comrades and I marched rapidly toward the Boche trenches, head lowered and throwing the body forward at each whistling of an obus. Now and again I raised my head, glanced around me quickly and then shrugged down into my shoulders.

Strangely, I had no fear, yet I knew that soon the figure of Death would be stalking among us. Always it rained, and this rain formed a mist through which the aeroplanes were indistinguishable. "That's going to make it bad for the artillery," thought I. On each side I saw our lines advancing, staggering, winding, tottering and again advancing. So, we stumbled forward for a hundred meters amongst a clattering riot of bursting obus of every caliber. Yet none near me had been wounded. Helas! How trivial was this vision to that which we were to later see.

Suddenly (I found myself among the first), I heard cries, "Forward, faster, run." Faster we ran, so that it was necessary to wait for one or two. The line must be straight to penetrate the first Boche trench.

Then indeed broke a hailstorm of iron. I saw my comrades coming up to me with heads lowered, I heard the spiteful tac-tac of the German machine guns (mitrailleuses) and, at the end of a few seconds, I remarked that we had before us at least ten mitrailleuses. I ran back quickly, my lieutenant was down, mortally stricken, among many other soldiers. Close to me another threw out his arms, wheeled around and fell. From all about me came cries. I was conscious of the reality. Before my eyes was unfolding one of the most terrible scenes of modern warfare.

All this last occurred in the space of two or three minutes. Thicker now the bullets rained around us. Comrades sank down beside me uttering always guttural cries.

The obus were beginning to burst above our heads. Always I advanced. A great hatred of the Boches surged through me and a fire of blind rage flashed into my being. Our first wave was fast becoming less dense. Many already would never answer again to the call, but I saw others coming up behind us and that gave me renewed confidence.

I was losing breath; the board which I was holding in the left hand prevented me from firing. I slackened my pace. Two comrades rejoined me; one had already fought a long campaign, the other, like myself, was in the first attack, and showed signs of fear, I thought. The first ran doggedly forward, superb, thinking of nothing. I had never seen the Boches in their first line of trenches; he had seen many. Coming up to me, he cried, "Have no fear, 'Mon petit gars,' and follow me; 'ça ira'!"

The second arrived and closed up with him; I did the same. There was no more sound of the mitrailleuses, so that I cried: "All goes well!" At that same moment, I felt a violent blow in the head, I wheeled and staggered, * * * I was blind ; a feeling of whirling fire spun through my brain * * * I was blind!

I thought myself lost and let my rifle fall. Then whispering a last adieu to my poor mother, already widowed by the war; a faint prayer to the Virgin, I fell.

How long did I lie there knowing nothing? I cannot tell. But the struggle must have raged tremendously around me. When at last I came to myself, I found myself mixed in a pile of other wounded lying at the bottom of a deep hole that had been made by a bursting obus.

I could see nothing, absolutely nothing, and I was bleeding profusely from the nose, mouth and forehead. There was hardly any pain. Continually, the obus burst around us. The German mitrailleuses never ceased their infernal chattering; ours remained mute; our mitrailleurs being nearly all killed or wounded.

About the hole to which I had been carried, the Corporal Brossire had rallied a few men to preserve us, if possible, from massacre at the hands of the enemy, in case they reached us. I remember that he placed upon me the dead body of a corporal as a protection from projectiles.

Many times the Boches tried to reach us, but they were always repulsed, grace to the courage of this Corporal Brossire who could always, in a tragic moment, find those words which put added courage into the hearts of his men. Wounded in the skull, he continued to command and to scorch with a glance those who spoke of retreat or surrender. "We will die here if we must," said he, "but never will I give up these wounded comrades."

The situation becomes more and more critical. After two hours of incessant and unequal fighting, the corporal and his men resign themselves to that beckoning figure of Death which has for so long been reaching toward us. They fire no more; their arms, grimed with mud, refuse to answer to the trigger. The Boches, in their turn advance in quick rushes; now, they have only thirty meters between themselves and us. "Don't stir," cries Brossire; "act as if dead, every one of you; they will pass attention, here they are,"

We wait, two, three, four seconds during which I can hear the pounding of my heart. What is happening? Suddenly one of our mitrailleuses makes itself heard behind us. It is at its maximum of speed and the bullets whistle above us, rushing to sow death among that advancing group.

A cry from the corporal, "Saved, mes enfants, it is Meyer; he is working for us." The brave Meyer, a sergeant mitrailleur, alone by his piece has in a few moments turned our terrible enemy.

Toward three o'clock I was found by a soldier who was carrying to the rear his wounded adjutant and who had found me in his path. Seeing me thus blind, he had offered to lead me to the rear before starting again for the front.

Once in our trenches, I was confided, with other wounded, to a party of Boche prisoners, who, under careful guard, carried us upon their back through the "boyaux" up to the first "Poste de Secours." Among these was a Bavarian who spoke French as well as I and who had not the grace to admit a defeat which now showed itself so certain, and who even dared to criticise our mode of attack, stating that we should be forever hated and despised by neutral nations when they would learn how terrible had been our bombardment.

I reached the ambulance very tired, twice I had fainted on the way and felt capable of nothing more. The morrow, I was in Châlons, where I was operated in the right eye, and later sent to the Ambulance at Juilly, where, at the hands of gentle American women, I received the tenderest care. On the 14th of October I was operated on and after a long treatment with many irrigations, I feel well now.

Here I end my story, in the course of which I have wished to forget no detail nor to imagine anything.

It will be a day of dullness for me when I will leave you and those ancient walls of Juilly, inside of which during my unhappiness, I found such beautiful days.

CHAPTER X.

THE TRIALS OF A MÉDECINE-CHEF.

The change from being a staff surgeon to Médecin-Chef had its advantages and drawbacks. Along with the authority suddenly imposed on one and the opportunity of running things as one thought best, this position brought with it responsibilities and the unenviable position of having everything disagreeable that arose put "up to the Médecin-Chef." The greatest drawback to the position is that one is deprived of the intimate contact with the poilus.

In the system of hospital management one man, the Médecin-Chef, is given full authority and made responsible for each and every department. This system has its advantage as the hospital is conducted by a medical man and the friction that often arises in civil hospitals between the medical staff and the office, is eliminated. At the same time a heavy task is imposed on the Médecin-Chef. He is responsible to the government for the welfare of the wounded entrusted to his care, must superintend the treatment and see that the military papers are properly filled out. Then there are the countless details of the surgical department, viz., the keeping up of supplies and equipment, the discipline of the hospital, the engaging of nurses, etc.

The housekeeping department comprises the supervision of the kitchen, store room, laundry, and the work of the house cleaners. Some of our food we buy in Paris and bring out in a camion. The meat and bread are delivered from the town of Dammartin, milk is purchased from a country dairyman, and butter, eggs, fresh vegetables and cheese we buy in the Saturday market at Meaux. Complications are constantly arising. The camion breaks down just as it is needed to haul supplies. The milk delivered is found to be sour and cannot be used. The turkeys were delivered at the hospital unplucked and the kitchen staff are sore because they have to pluck them. The poilus complain that the meat was not properly cooked and upon interviewing the cook he blames the coal, which at $20 a ton contains a goodly amount of dirt and rock. Some of the nurses refuse to eat rabbit and kid after they discover what they are. Two of the cook's assistants have a fight and the row has to be straightened out. Then the pump breaks down unexpectedly and for two days all the water has to be carried upstairs in buckets. A fire breaks out in the laundry, burns up a lot of the wash and a laundress has a hysterical fit.

Splints and fracture boards are needed and the village carpenter and blacksmith must have the appliances explained to them. A stove in the theatre smokes and it is found that the smoke stack has two elbows and doesn't draw properly. No stove piping is to be had ready made and it will take two weeks to have it made in Paris. Milk is being spilled on the stairways as it is being carried to the wards. By close watch two culprits are caught and sufficiently admonished. Telephone communication is suddenly cut off without any explanation and remains cut off in spite of a telegram of protest. We have gotten so used to having our electric lights go out that we are prepared for it and have a plentiful supply of candles and lanterns.

After such a day with perhaps half a dozen operations, the Médecin-Chef's labors are not over. There are the bills and vouchers to look over, as the Médecin-Chef has to approve of the expenditure of every franc.

The wounded nearly always arrive at night, usually several hours later than the time announced. At first we used to wait up for them but found it was a better plan to rest and be called by the night orderlies when the first ambulance arrived. The Médecin-

Chef then had to superintend the job, see that the blessés are properly handled, undressed and bathed, look over their injuries, assign them to the different wards and decide whether immediate operations are necessary.

A trip to Paris was often a mad rush to get things attended to. A day in Paris might pass like this: An effort to arrange that some of our heavier supplies would go out by train encountered at once "red-tape" and uncertainty of train service. Two hours were spent trying to get a dozen beds. After going a long way to a wholesale place and choosing the bed we wanted, found that it was only a sample. They said they couldn't make any more because their workers were mobilized and it is difficult to get iron. The Germans hold most of the iron mines. Then went miles across Paris suburbs to order some iron tables and by chance landed on a bed manufactory. It was a disreputable looking place but the proprietor agreed to make beds at thirty francs each. Then to the instrument maker to get the surgical knives which had been left there to be sharpened and found that they had been sent by mistake to Ris-Orangis. No screws for Lane plates to be had but they could be made by hand for a franc apiece and it would take a week to make six. The proprietor explained that they had been in the habit of getting such things from Germany. This is a sample of how difficult it is to get things. I have to hurry to a meeting of the Juilly Committee at the American Ambulance at Neuilly. Mr. Robert Bacon is there and a talk with him inspires me to greater effort.

Arriving back at Juilly after dark my troubles were not over for the day. Some convalescents were to be evacuated and three of them were intoxicated. We had remarkably little trouble with the soldiers drinking. Considering the hardships and sufferings they had been through, an occasional lapse would not have been strange, and the absence of drinking showed the fine discipline in the French army.

This offense of being intoxicated had then to be thoroughly investigated. The next morning the three delinquents, looking very sheepish, are called into my office and admonished. They all confess their fault, were sorry and were pardoned. It appeared that they got the liquor in a little village a mile away. We went to the village and accused the woman in charge of the wineshop of selling liquor to the soldiers. She denied it but when confronted with one of the soldiers then tried to put it off on her fifteen-year-old daughter. The mayor was then hunted up but as he was absent, we called on the acting mayor. He was a little peasant disturbed at his noonday meal of a savory ragout and salad. In reply to our complaint, he agreed that it was a grave offense and would act as we wanted. What did we want him to do? Close the "bistro" for eight days. All right, he would do so if we would write out a complaint and an order of closure. So back to the hospital we went and wrote out the two papers, and then back to the mayor's. "All right, I will attend to it tomorrow as today is Sunday and perhaps there will be customers there." "So much the better," he was told, "and it must be attended to at once." But then he wasn't dressed. No matter, we would be glad to wait and drive him over in our auto. So at last it was attended to. The mayor dressed, went along with us, gave the orders forbidding any sales for eight days. The incident is closed but had a salutary effect on all concerned.

France has ever been famous for her good cooking and the stress of war has not broken down this admirable characteristic. To a Frenchman meal time is an institution to be enjoyed with a zest and a touch of the artistic. The soldiers are well fed and, except in time of heavy action, have plenty of well-cooked food. Some of the 4000 hospitals used for wounded soldiers at times have difficulty in providing certain food for the wounded. Chickens and butter are sometimes difficult to obtain or are beyond the reach of the hospital's finances, but bread, eggs, milk, vegetables and meat, in moderate quantities, are usually available.

The prices of food, transposed from kilograms and francs into pounds and cents, that we paid in 1915-16 were:

Beef and mutton, 28 cents a pound.

Chickens, about $1.35 each.

Rabbits, 75 cents apiece.

Bread, from 3 to 4 cents a pound.

Butter, 35 cents a pound.

Eggs, 35 cents a dozen.

Potatoes, 2 cents a pound.

Beet sugar, 10 cents a pound. Later the price went to 24 cents and sugar was difficult to obtain in large quantities.

Coffee, 38 cents a pound.

Milk, 5 cents a quart.

Rice, 8 cents a pound.

The total daily cost of feeding each individual in the hospital, patients and staff, was 56 cents a day.

Chapter XI.

Holidays and Festivals.

On Thanksgiving Day we were as American as could be and the staff celebrated the day by having roast turkey stuffed with chestnuts and a huge pumpkin pie. As Thanksgiving day did not mean anything to the poilus we concentrated our efforts in preparing Christmas and New Year's entertainments for them.

The French winter is nothing to be proud of. The first week in December it was so cold that some of the soldiers in the trenches had their feet frozen. By the middle of December it was too warm for an overcoat. By Christmas time it was freezing again. There was little snow, but it rained nearly every day. It grew dark at 3:30 in the afternoon and our lighting bills increased considerably. Things are rather quiet in the bad weather, and apparently the two lines of trenches settled down for the winter, each one with the feeling that the other is unable to break through their line.

The Christmas celebration was a great success. The wards were decorated with strings of colored paper running from the walls to the electric lights, the walls were decorated with wreaths of ivy and bunches of holly and mistletoe were hung in the windows. The wooden frameworks for suspending broken limbs were festooned with ivy. Altogether the effect was very pretty.

A ward decorated for Christmas

On Christmas eve the boys from the college sang for the blessés. Some of them had very sweet voices. They had a small but heavy organ which they carried from one ward to another and one of the professors played the accompaniments, making a goodly number of discords. Nevertheless, the soldiers enjoyed the music hugely.

On Christmas morning there was much handshaking and exchange of "Bonne Noël." In every ward there was a tree decorated with imitation snow, tinsel and candles. Every soldier received a bag containing simple gifts as writing pads, socks, pipes, candy, etc. A huge Ambulance driver made a realistic Santa Claus and amused the blessés as he distributed the presents.

Our wounded colonel made a gracious speech, which one of the staff took down in shorthand. Of course it suffers from being translated, but is worth recording.

"Ladies and Gentlemen of the American Ambulance of Juilly:

"In the name of my wounded comrades and in my own name, I beg to thank you for your delicate thought in giving to us the illusion of our absent family by this Christmas celebration. I desire also to express to you our appreciation of the devotion and science of the doctors and the professional skill and devoted care of the nurses who have carried to the bedside of the wounded the charm of their grace and their smiles. Thus have you lightened our sufferings and saved most of us, myself among them. I certainly represent all the wounded when I say that we shall never forget the devoted care which you have given us. I ask you to applaud 'un triple ban' in honor of the Ambulance." (Here the assembly followed the Colonel's suggestion and clapped hands in the French fashion.)

"Christmas recalls to us very sweet memories. As children we placed our slippers in the chimney place and prayed to the Christ child or to St. Nicholas to bring us the toys that we wanted. The next morning, with our happy parents, we had the joy of finding the gifts that we longed for. Later on in life, we have enjoyed the customary midnight gaiety, and Christmas has always been the fête day for the children and family.

"We are very appreciative that the staff of the ambulance has created such a family atmosphere for our Christmas day.

"As these days go by we must remember that our task is not yet achieved and that we should by our patience and will hasten our recovery so that those of us who can, and that will be most of us, shall engage again in the unfinished combat. On this question, you must believe, no matter what you hear, that victory is certain and that in the months to come we shall drive back the Boches. We shall impose the terms of peace, a victorious peace and prevent them from again committing their crimes. You can be certain of the future that nous les aurons."

The dinner was extra good with turkey and cranberry sauce in plenty. There was music by local talent and by some professionals who came out from Paris. A cinema rented for the occasion gave some excellent moving pictures and there were games for

44

the convalescents, as bean bags and ninepins. Fortunately there were no very sick patients, so all could enjoy themselves.

On Christmas morning I was called into my old ward and presented with a handsome smoking set. At the same time one of the blessés read in a loud voice the following speech.

"Je viens au nom de mes camarades remercier Madame et Monsieur le Docteur Judd et ses distingués collaborateurs des soins dévoués dont vous nous entourez. Mr. le docteur vous avez quitté vos blessés avec regret. Vous, qui les soignez avec la sollicitude d'une mère; vous, qui veniez pendant certains nuits apporter votre science à plusieurs d'entre nous, vous étiez un père pour tous. Elevé au grade de médecin-chef, l'inquiétude de ne plus recevoir vos soins nous attriste. Heureusement votre successeur se montre d'un dévouement à toute épreuve et tous nous remercions et nous nous écrions ensemble.

"Vive la France!

"Vive l'Amérique."

At the same time they presented L. with a beautiful bouquet of roses.

New Year's day is highly esteemed by the soldiers, and we had the same sort of a celebration without the trees. The presence of 600 soldiers just back from the trenches made quite a little excitement in the village.

On Toussaints day the soldiers' graves in the little village cemetery were decorated. We made up a procession, doctors, nurses, ambulance drivers and convalescents and marched to the cemetery, the nurses carrying wreaths. The French show a marked reverence for the dead. The soldiers' graves are close together, but each one is marked with a little white cross giving the soldier's name and military station. The Algerians' graves have a foot board with a star and crescent on it and the graves are placed obliquely heading towards Mecca. Graves are scattered thickly over parts of France and no one has been allowed to remove the bodies of their relatives. That must wait until after the war.

At Commencement time there were exercises in the College. A play was cleverly carried off. The French are born actors. Monseigneur Marabeau, the bishop of Meaux, graced the occasion with his presence. He is a successor to the famous Bossuet and is a striking personality. Tall and of commanding presence he is every inch a leader. He made the rounds of the hospital and shook hands with every poilu, inquiring of their home town and gave each one a "jolly." He must have traveled extensively in France, because he seemed to have a bon mot for everyone, making jokes about their districts and causing many a laugh.

The French priests have certainly shown up well in the war. We hear that there are 8,000 in the army. There is a heavy burden on those who are not in the trenches, as the labor of caring for the sick and poor has greatly increased. The soldiers as a rule are devout Catholics and most of them go to mass when they are able. The war has brought about a spiritual awakening in France. Widows and mothers who have lost their husbands and sons turn to the church for comfort and strong men facing death look to the church for spiritual strength to meet the great test. The director of the college is a militant churchman, and is with the army at Salonica, where he has been wounded and promoted for bravery.

July 14th, the French great national holiday, was one of the most inspiring days we have lived through. We learned that there was going to be a parade of the Allies' troops, so we came in to Paris to see it. Our view point was the roof of the Hotel Crillon, looking down on the Place de la Concorde. The square was black with people, leaving only an open space for the troops to march through. Down along the Champs Elysées they came, over the spot where the guillotine stood, through the Place, past the obelisk and up the rue Royale. All the Allies were represented. There were of course the poilus with their steel helmets and blue uniforms, foot soldiers, bicycle corps, cavalry and Algerian troops and an artillery detachment with the famous soixante-quinze. English, Scotch, Irish, Canadian, Australian, New Zealand and Indian troops represented Great Britain. A Belgian company was there and Russians, the biggest men of all. Italian soldiers with their waving feather plumes made a natty appearance. Even Servia was represented by a few troops and the Annamites from Franco-China.

The crowd went wild and cheered themselves hoarse and the sight was inspiring to everyone. There was not an American onlooker who did not have the feeling in his heart that our boys in khaki should be there marching along with the French and British and the others, and that perhaps they would be by the next anniversary of the fall of the Bastille.

Chapter XII.

Senlis.

One of the many acts of barbarism committed by the Germans which have arrayed most of the civilized world against them has been the destruction of unprotected and helpless towns and the shooting of civilians. In Belgium and in Northern France there has always been the same old excuse that the civilians had fired on their troops. This has been proved over and over again to be false. In other cases shots were fired but they were fired by accidental or intended discharge of German rifles or Belgian and French soldiers on the village outskirts had fired on the enemy. Even if in some isolated instances civilians had fired on the Germans (which is not admitted and has not been authenticated) there is absolutely no justification for the wholesale burning of houses and murder of innocent men, women and children.

Senlis suffered such a fate and the story of her sufferings may be cited as a typical example of the German policy of "frightfulness." What senseless barbarism to thus try and intimidate the French! No people has greater love of country and home than the French, and Germany's barbarism and inhumanity, far from terrorising the French, made them all the more determined in the defense of their homes and country.

Those who know this part of France will remember Senlis as one of the most charming towns of this region. Situated near the forest of Chantilly, the wooded country furnishes excellent stag hunting and the chief hostelry of the town is named "L'hôtel du Grand Cerf." The interesting little arena, walls and towers are among the best relics of Roman rule in Northern France, while the old chateau of Henri IV and the splendid cathedral furnish a wealth of sightseeing to a visitor.

Nowadays the visitor sees first the railway station burned; only a shell of wall stands, over which waves the tricolor. Nearly all the houses lining the rue de la République have been burned, also the St. Martin quarter.

Some of the walls standing give evidence of former splendor as is the case of the Palais de Justice and some of the large private residences. Those that suffered most were the humbler dwellings of the bourgeois. Even the hospital was not spared. We saw the wall riddled with bullet holes of the machine guns. The bullets had not touched the crucifix on the wall but had surrounded it in a remarkable manner. We heard from the sweet-faced sister how they were caring not only for French wounded but for German soldiers when the hospital was fired on. In the unmolested quarter is a small house on the door of which is written in chalk, "Gute Leute—Bitte Schoenen." The inmates have disappeared long since. Had this anything to do with Germany's very complete spy system? The writing is still there and serves the purpose of a warning and reminder.

On September 1, 1914, the sound of cannon was heard in the near distance, but the inhabitants had no idea of their impending fate. A number of people had already departed, but the Mayor and city officials remained at their post. On September 2nd the sound became louder and a large part of the population fled, some on foot, some on bicycles, others in wagons. The stores began to close and excitement increased. Soon some French troops appeared, fighting in retreat, and crossed the city in the direction of Paris. The inhabitants quickly became aware of the proximity of the Germans when shells began to fall, killing a few people. At four o'clock the German troops of Von Kluck's army appeared, marching through the streets in two columns. At the Mairie they demanded the "bourgomaester" and the Mayor, Eugène Odent, presented himself, and he was at once marched off to the Hôtel du Grand Cerf, where the Germans established their headquarters. The French troops who had passed through Senlis in retreat had posted themselves on the outskirts towards Chantilly and fired on the advance guards of the Germans. The mayor was then faced with the accusation that the inhabitants had fired on the Germans and this he denied vehemently, as they had no arms and had been instructed to offer no resistance. Then followed the inhuman crimes of the Germans as a punishment for the legitimate attack of the French rear guard. The Mayor and six citizens seized at hazard in the streets, were taken to the suburb of Chamant and, without any trial or opportunity to say farewell to their families, were shot forthwith. Here are the names of the victims:

Eugène Odent, mayor, 59 years of age;

Arthur Rigualt, stone cutter, 61 years of age;

Romand Aubert, tanner, 52 years of age;

Jean Pommier, laborer, 67 years of age;

Jean Barbier, driver, 66 years of age;

Arthur Cottrau, dish washer, 17 years of age;

Pierre Dewert, chauffeur, 45 years of age.

Several citizens, including Madame Painchaux and her five year old child, were seized and forced to march before the German soldiers down the rue de la République, where most of them were shot down by French bullets before the French soldiers on the edge of the forest ceased firing.

The rage of the Germans upon meeting any opposition knew no bounds, and a good part of Senlis was set in flames. To burn a defenseless town they were well prepared with incendiary apparatus, bombs and grenades. A hundred and four houses were burned and it was with the greatest difficulty that the Archbishop Dourlent received the concession that the entire town would not be burned.

"They have fired on us and officers and soldiers have been killed. See, this is the first chastisement, this street that is burning. Tonight Senlis will undergo the same fate and tomorrow not a house will be left standing."

The archbishop overwhelmed at these words replied,

"It cannot be possible that you would commit this crime. They have not fired on you. It is the French army that has been firing on your troops."

"Soldiers against soldiers," replied the officer, "c'est la guerre, but civilians and priests fired on us at Louvain in the street and from the church tower. Here the same thing has happened."

The priest replied vehemently, "I do not know what happened at Louvain, but no one has fired from the cathedral tower here. I alone have the key to the tower since the beginning of hostilities, and I have given it to no one. This morning I climbed up into the tower to see where the fighting was going on so as to be able to direct those of my parishioners who wished to flee. You don't suppose that I am able to carry a machine gun into the tower? I am telling you the truth and will take my oath to it."

The murdering of the Mayor and six inoffensive citizens, the use of men, women and children as a shield for their troops against French bullets, the destruction of a large part of the town by fire did not satisfy the furor Teutonica. Pillage remained for the brute appetite. Houses were broken open, cellars ransacked and they satiated their thirst in drunken orgies. No one was safe from these frenzied Huns. The story of Simon the tobacconist is typical of what happened. On the second of September, towards the middle of the afternoon, a dozen soldiers entered his shop. "A boire," they commanded in their drunken rage. Simon hurried to serve them and, while some of them drank, others helped themselves to tobacco and the small stock of groceries. "A boire, encore et toujours." There was no more wine drawn, so Simon sent his father-in-law and assistant to the cellar for more. "More wine and quickly," and as the service seemed too slow they seized the three men violently crying, "You fired at us." Simon protested that he had not fired and besides that he had never had a weapon in his house. He had no chalice to protest further as he was placed against the wall and shot. The assistant escaped, the father-in-law was one of those placed in front of the German troops as a protection and was mortally wounded. Poor Simon's shop stands there today, that is the ruins of it, marked by the legend on a board "Débit Simon."

And so on, other stories could be told of the killing of innocent civilians.

The ruins of Senlis, the graves of innocent victims and the memories of those frightful days remain as in many a town of Belgium and Northern France an irrefutable record of German criminal wantonness.

CHAPTER XIII.

THE BATTLEFIELD OF THE MARNE.

The battle of the Marne was stupendous. Visitors who see a part of the battle field by way of Meaux gain but a small idea of its extent but a good idea of its intensity. It was in the region of Meaux that a critical phase of the battle developed when General Manoury's Sixth Army held and began to turn the flank of Von Kluck's First German Army.

The line of battle extended from Nanteuil almost to Verdun, a distance of about 120 miles. The battle lasted from the 5th to the 12th of September, 1914. The distance from the northern to the southern edge of the battlefield may be said to be roughly 50 miles, so that the battle field area may be estimated to cover an area of 6,000 square miles. The battlefield is historic ground. Fourteen centuries ago the invading Huns had been driven back on the field of Châlons. On the day that the French first declared a republic, in 1792, the invaders had been repulsed at Valmy. Napoleon executed some of his brilliant exploits on these same fields.

As regards the number of troops engaging in the battle an official announcement has not as yet been given. The army corps and divisions engaged are known but the impossibility of knowing what casualties had occurred since the beginning of the war, only makes an estimate possible. On the Allies side it is probable that 700,000 men were under General Joffre's orders, It is generally believed, except by the German public, that the Germans were in superior numbers, probably over a million. Compared with Napoleon's time, at the battle of Waterloo there were 60,000 French and 70,000 allies engaged. In modern times at the battle of Mukden there were 270,000 Russian troops and 280,000 Japanese, while in the greatest battle of our Civil War there were about 150,000 troops on both sides.

The first shot of the battle apparently was fired from a German battery at Monthyon at noon on September 5th. Paris lies but twenty-two miles away, and on a clear day the Eiffel tower may be seen from the Monthyon hill top.

The town of Meaux narrowly escaped as the battle reached to its very gates. The bridges connecting the thirteenth century mills with the river banks were blown up to delay the German advance, but the town itself was only slightly damaged by shell fire.

49

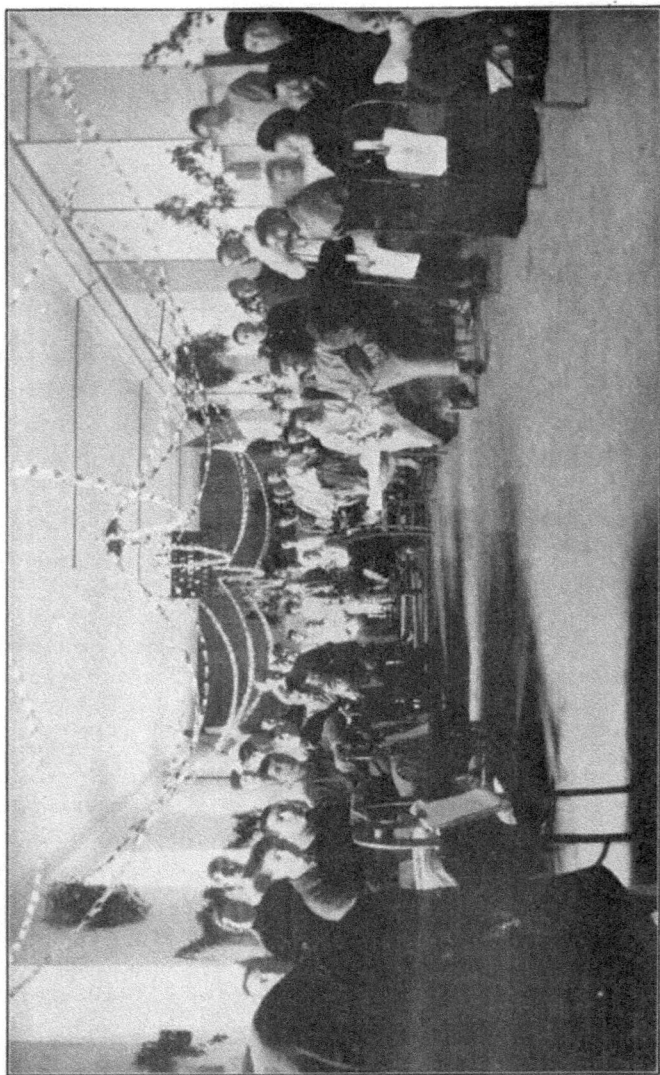

A ward decorated for Christmas.

Spread out to the north and east of Meaux lies a rich, agricultural plain on each side of the Marne valley. The villages scattered over this plain show signs of heavy fighting. Houses have been demolished by shell fire and walls are pock marked by bullets. Barcy, Chambry, Chauconin, Etrépilly, Marcilly and Etavigny are all historic names.

At Chambry the Germans had transformed the cemetery into a fortress by piercing the walls with loop-holes for their machine guns. From this stronghold they were brilliantly driven out by the Zouaves. The numerous bullet marks showing on the walls, monuments and tombs of the cemetery give some idea of how fierce the fighting must have been.

Scattered over the fields are hundreds and thousands of graves, each one marked with a little white cross, many with a small French flag and some with the dead soldier's red cap pathetically resting on top of the cross.

The places where the French threw themselves against the invaders in bayonet charges are easy to find as here the graves are thick. Scattered here and there are isolated graves near some village where a badly wounded man perhaps tried to crawl for help and bled to death on the way.

Hung to the little posts enclosing the graves are seen here and there wide mouthed bottles containing written messages. Within these bottles one can read a message from a mother or wife begging for anyone who can to give them information about their missing son or husband. Rarely will their aching hearts learn anything about their loved one. He has been buried unmarked, a shapeless and unidentified mass, or a shell explosion has wiped him out completely.

On a hill commanding a view of the surrounding country is the farm of Champfleury. Here Von Kluck had his headquarters for eight days and saw that the battle was lost, retreat was necessary to save what was left and Germany's dream of world conquest was shattered. The farm house has been repaired since the Germans left it, but it shows numerous scars of bullets and shell fire. The proprietor told us that he left in his automobile for Paris as the Germans were seen coming over the hill from the north. There was no hesitation or hunting for suitable headquarters. The desirable sites were apparently well known. The proprietor, of the wealthy farmer class, had a good wine cellar, which he found thoroughly demolished on his return. In the front grounds stands a cherry tree with an iron chair wedged securely among its branches. This seat must have commanded a fine view of the battle for a staff officer or perhaps Von Kluck himself. On a wall and on a table top are written some pleasantries in German script with allusions to the good times they had had with champagne and billiards and regrets at leaving. These writings have not been effaced, nor has the billiard room, battered and smashed, been changed from the condition in which it was found on the return of the owner.

Beyond Champfleury is the farm of Poligny, very effectually burned by the Germans. The large wheat hangar was used by the enemy as a funeral pyre for 2000 of their dead, and its twisted girders have fallen in on a mass of ashes, broken tiles and melted bones. In this region the Germans used a number of hangars for the same purpose, perhaps because there was no time to bury their dead, perhaps because they did not want their opponents to know the extent of their losses. Frightened peasants who were hiding in their cellars tell of shrieks of dying men who were thrown into the fire.

At Etavigny, where there was heavy fighting, village children presented us with handfuls of shrapnel balls picked up in the fields. The church was badly damaged by shells and lying at the portal is the church bell, rent in twain. Among some blood stained straw strewn over the floor we picked up some exploded cartridges.

Beyond Etavigny, where the Germans made a stand, is a long line of trench now overgrown with grass. There were empty tin cans, bits of clothing and leather to be seen scattered about. Our chauffeur told us that on a previous visit he had found a German boot attached to what was once a leg, sticking out of the ground.

The booming of the cannon towards the east, the little tri-color flags waving over the graves scattered among the growing crops, the shell marked ruined villages, the rolling plains stretching in every direction, are bound to produce in the visitor's mind the question, "Why did not the German army sweep on as they had through Belgium and Northern France and capture Paris?" "How was it that this powerful machine with forty years of preparation was stopped and driven back?"

Among other problems, the military writers for centuries to come will be kept busy on the explanation of the battle of the Marne.

In an analysis of the reasons for the defeat of the world-grasping German plan, the vitalizing moral forces of the armies will ever be preëminent. Napoleon said that "in war the moral is to the physical as three is to one."

The French soldiers were fighting in defense of their country, their homes, wives and children. The British soldier thought of homes a few miles across the channel. The German soldier was fighting a war of aggression, carnage, destruction of innocent towns and civilians. The vain glory of hacking through Belgium and Northern France with superior force, the lust of blood and slaughter could not stand against the moral forces of patriotism and sacrifice that opposed them. Joffre well knew the French soldier in his famous order of the day when he said, "Une troupe qui ne pourra plus avancer devra, coûte que coûte, garder le terrain conquis et se faire tuer plutôt que de reculer."

CHAPTER XIV.

AVIATORS.

Early in the spring an aviation training camp was established at Plessis-Belleville, about five miles from Juilly. A wheat field was cleared off, huge hangars were erected and, in a few days, a great number of aeroplanes made their appearance. There were a variety of makes, from the heavy, slow Farnam to the rapid Nieuport.

We were officially notified that we were now attached to the organization as the surgical hospital, and we did not have long to wait for our patients. Almost on the first

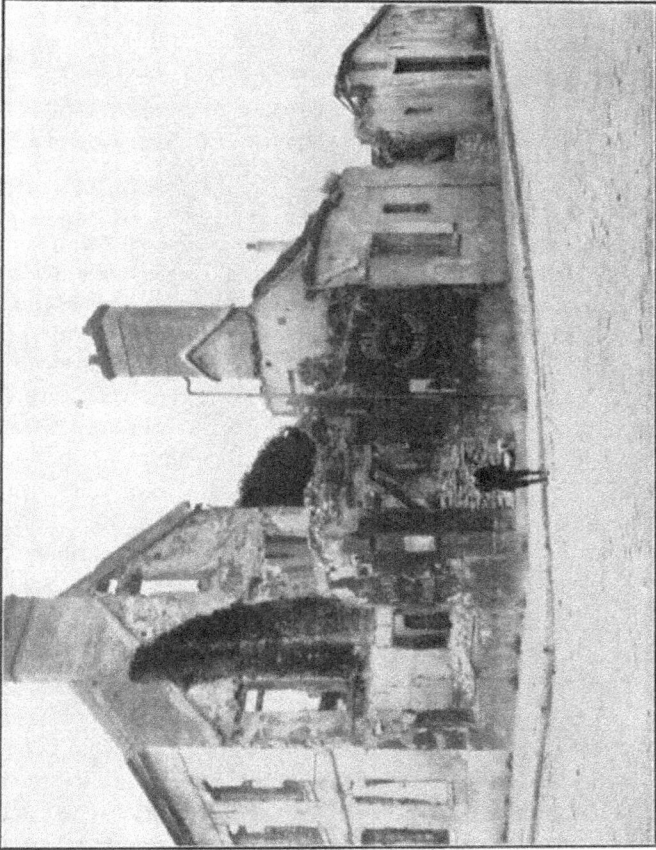

German "Kultur" at Senlis.

day an aeroplane fell from a great height and two aviators were brought in with broken skulls, one to die in a few hours, the other to recover, partly paralyzed, after a long illness.

The aviators are a superior lot of men. First, they have to pass strict physical tests, and also they are for the most part men of superior education. Some of them are descendants of the old nobility and still cherish inherited titles. Some speak English well and have traveled in America. The flyers are young men, as older men, over thirty, are considered to be too cautious. The French say that to be an aviator a man has to be a little peculiar—that a normal, sane man does not make a good flyer.

Accidents are frequent, five in one day. They are of varying severity. One man got too near a propeller and had half his scalp torn off. Broken legs and arms. are common. One poor fellow was high up in the air when his machine caught fire and he was picked up a charred corpse.

An afternoon at the flying field is a great sight. There are dozens of aeroplanes ascending and descending. Others are soaring around in the heavens at great heights. The aviators dress in a variety of uniforms, which seem to be chosen according to personal taste, as there is no fixed uniform. For cold weather they have shaggy coats of animal skins. The headquarters are located in Prince Radziwill's beautiful château at Ermenonville. The building is surrounded by a moat in medieval style. On a small island in a nearby lake is the empty tomb of Rousseau, where the famous philosopher was buried before his remains were transferred to the Pantheon. The Germans were here in September, 1914, but limited their depredations to smashing in a few closets and bureaus. Some of the servants of the château gleaned that the Germans counted on returning after Paris was captured, in order to enjoy the hunting for which Ermenonville is famous.

After the aviation field had been in use some months word passed around the Ambulance that there were some American boys there in training. We hoped to see them and were delighted one day, shortly before they left for the front, to have a call from Thaw, Prince, McConnell and Rockwell. They were a fine lot of fellows with the quiet modesty of brave men who have done something worth while but do not boast about it. They are held in high esteem and admired by their French comrades, and it seemed as if there could be no better recognition of their bravery and skill. We were sorry not to see Victor Chapman. The French say he is very daring. Norman Prince is a nephew of Dr. Morton Prince of Boston, a well known alienist, and is a Harvard graduate. He is said to have originated the American Squadron as an organization. Thaw is a Yale man and has served in the Foreign Legion. He is about 25 but looks much older. Rockwell was also in the Foreign Legion. He is a Southerner and is tall and handsome. McConnell is also a Southerner but looks as if he might come from New England. Thaw and McConnell are powerfully built, Rockwell is slender and Prince is short and stocky. There is a quiet air of determination and devotion about these men that makes every one of us Americans feel proud of our fellow country-men.

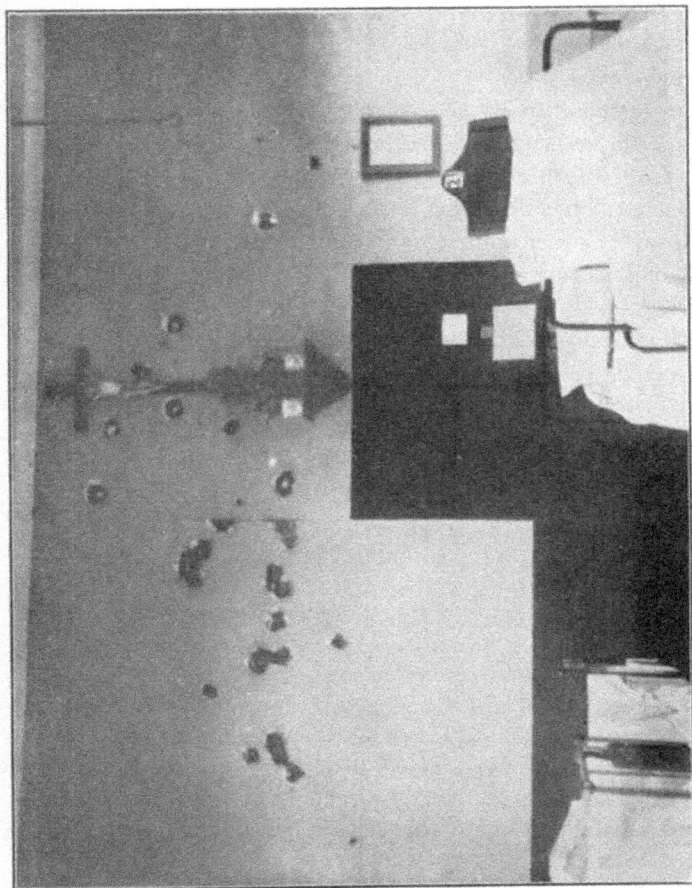

The crucifix in the hospital at Senlis, surrounded by bullet holes made by German guns.

We said good-by to them with sadness, feeling that it was perhaps good-by and not au revoir. Alas, our forebodings were too true. A few months later only Thaw is left. Rockwell, Prince and McConnell have fallen on the field of honor.

Well are these heroes worthy of the words of Alan „Seeger, the brilliant young poet of the Foreign Legion:

"Some there were
Who, not unmindful of the antique debt
Came back the generous path of Lafayette.
Yet sought they neither recompense nor praise,
Nor to be mentioned in another breath
Than their blue coated comrades whose great days
It was their pride to share—ay, share even to the death!
Nay, rather, France to you they rendered thanks
(Seeing they came for honor not for gain)
Who, opening to them your glorious ranks,
Gave them that grand occasion to excel,
That chance to live the life most free from stain
And that rare privilege of dying well."

CHAPTER XV.

INCIDENTS AND OBSERVATIONS.

We soon learned that there are several ways of speaking French. Our blessés came from almost every part of France, and as our ears became accustomed to the French sounds, we learned to tell in a general way from what part of France our soldiers came. The southerners who sounded the mute "e" and the Bretons, were almost unmistakable. Our "Henri IV" from Beam spoke in such a jerky manner that he was understood with difficulty by his comrades. He always called potatoes "potate" instead of "pomme de terre."

One little Breton who used to make a living by sailing to Dundee with loads of onions, spoke English with a Scotch accent and was nicknamed "Scottie." It was amusing to hear him talk, partly French and partly with his strong Scotch accent. He was shy at first, but gradually became conscious of his linguistic accomplishments, until one day when he was called on for a menial service by one of his comrades, announced that he was "the interpreter for the nurses."

After a while we learned that the soldiers use a good many words not to be found in any standard dictionary. In fact there is almost a new trench language, l'argot des tranchées. One has to learn some of it if he is going to understand what is going on. Paris is usually referred to as "Panam" or "Pantruche." The canned meat of the trench ration is "singe," coffee is "jus," wine is "pinard." A comrade is a "poteau" or "pote." A wine-shop is a "bistro" and so on. The origin of the word "poilu" is not

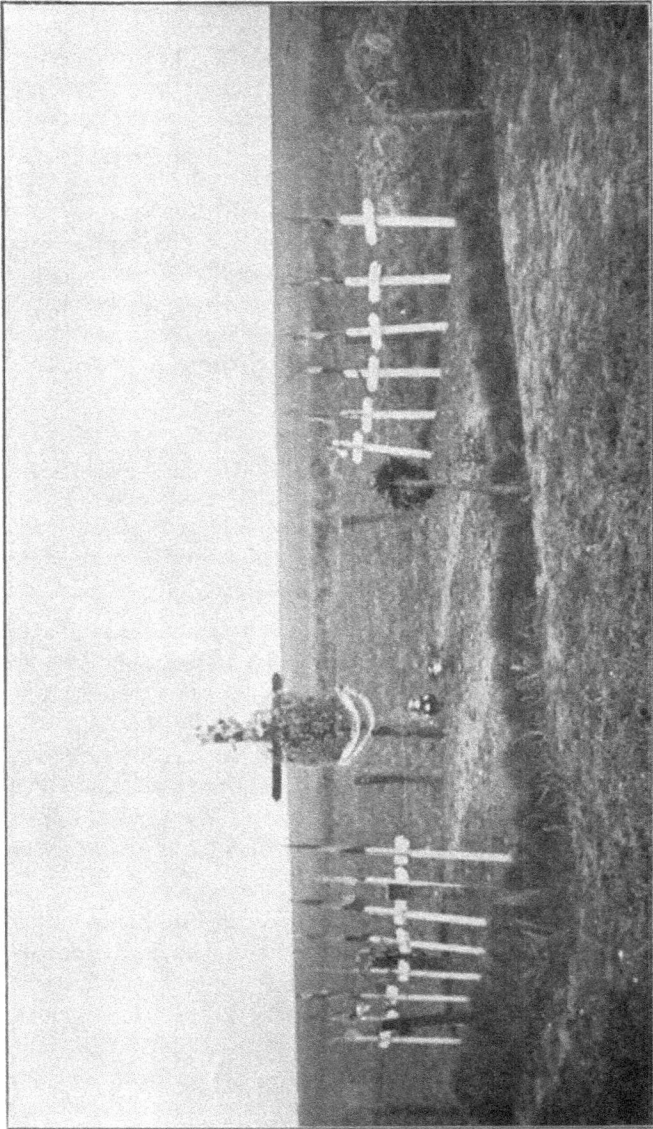

Where an officer and fourteen of his men are buried on the battlefield of the Marne.

settled. Some say it comes from the whiskered appearance of the soldiers on their return home on leave, others that it was a term applied to Napoleon's brigadiers on account of their large hair helmets. At any rate the term has come to stay, not only in French writings but in English.

One who has worked among French wounded cannot but be impressed with the absence of personal hatred shown by the French soldier against the Germans. They hate the things the Germans stand for, the invasion and devastation of peaceful countries, the destruction of unprotected towns,. the massacre of unoffending men, women and children, the use of gas and liquid fire in war-, fare, but it was rare to find any expression of hatred against the German soldier. In battle the French soldier fights like a man with a noble heritage in defense of his country and family, and it is well known that the Germans will not stand against them in a bayonet charge. But once the wounded German comes into his hands he is treated with the natural magnanimity of the race in the spirit of Bayard. The American Ambulance drivers tell us that they are instructed to carry badly wounded Germans to the rear while the French wounded lie there and await their turn.

I saw at Creil a little tow-headed Saxon prisoner in a hospital ward with twenty or more French soldiers. He received the same food as they did, laughed and joked with them, played cards and it was hard to realize that he was a prisoner. With the Major's permission I had a little conversation with him. He said he didn't know what they were fighting for and that he wished the war was over so that he could go home to his family—that he was called out and had to go with the army or be shot.

The French soldiers are a wonderfully happy lot of men. As soon as they are well enough, they enjoy life, relish their meals, play games, read, sing, listen to the graphophone, make rings out of pieces of shells and other trinkets, or walk around the park. Those who are laid up for a long time with a bad fracture, weave baskets or make shawls on a wooden frame. It was rare to see one idle. The men who come from the invaded districts, who have not seen or heard from their wives and children for months or years, have a different look in their eyes. It is a sad and thoughtful look. Woe betide any German who stands in front of them in a bayonet charge!

The French are fond of ceremony and their ceremonies of decorating soldiers are carried out in such a dignified and touching manner that they are inspiring. I shall never forget the first decoration that I saw. In the little square in front of the college; two companies of troops assembled. The troops were composed of territorials, old fellows, gray-haired and bald-headed—the country's last reserve. The soldiers formed a hollow square and presented arms, the bugles and trumpets sounded and a wounded one-armed soldier stepped forward into the center of the square, his checks red with excitement and his remaining hand twitching with nervous exhilaration.

The Colonel then read a recital of the soldier's deeds of valor, signed by Joffre, pinned the two decorations on the soldier's breast and kissed him on both cheeks. The trumpets sounded, the troops marched around the square and we all congratulated the proud soldier on receiving the Croix de Guerre and Médaille Militaire. We saw quite a number of decorations. When we had a lot of wounded from Verdun,

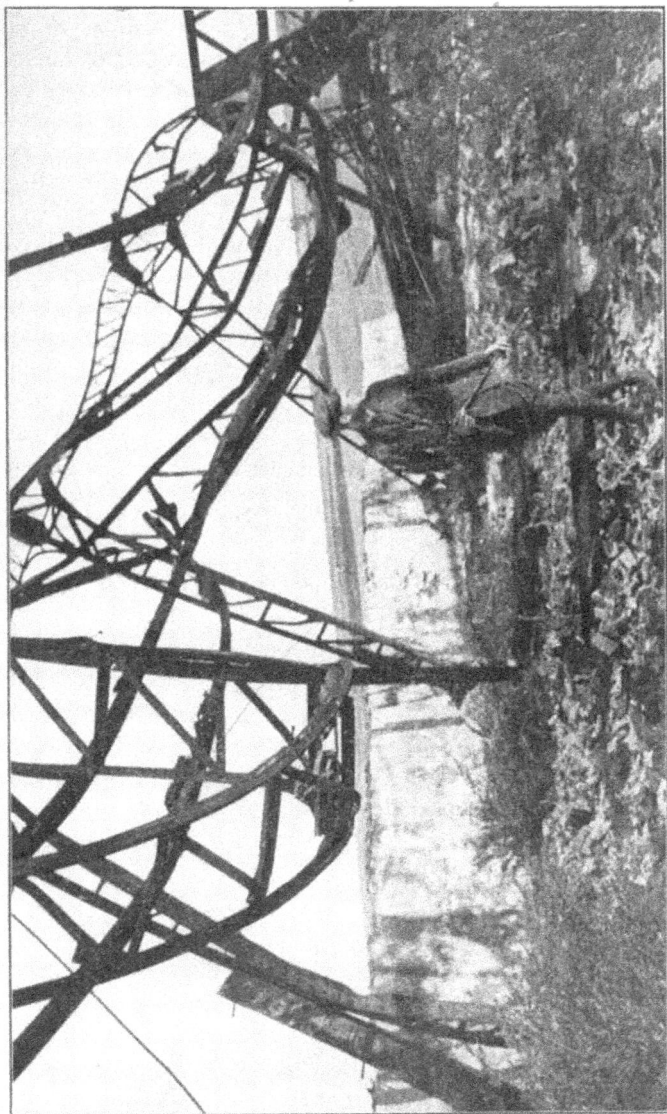

Where the Germans burned two thousand dead at Poligny.

sixteen men were decorated at one ceremony and the embrace on both cheeks had changed to a handshake. We had the feeling that every man who fought at Verdun was a hero and should be decorated.

The soldier's funeral is sad and there is such simplicity and pathos that we were always affected, but came away with the feeling that the soldier had done a big and noble thing in giving his life for his country. The funeral processions started at the hospital and filed across the little square to the village church. The blessés were there, everyone who could make it—some on crutches, others with arms in splints and heads swathed in bandages. The village priest intoned the service assisted in the responses by the choir, consisting of one old man and a nun who played the church organ. The ceremony over, all who could walked to the cemetery on the edge of the village. The coffin was usually carried by a detail of artillerymen from the neighboring post. At the cemetery the coffin was deposited by the side of the freshly dug grave, the priest chanted the ritual, each one in turn sprinkled holy water on the bier and the crowd departed leaving flowers on the coffin. No salute was fired, as no powder is wasted. The booming of cannon towards Soissons always brought to us the reality of war.

If the relatives of the dead soldier were present they always stood at the gate of the cemetery and shook hands with and thanked each one of us as we passed by.

The poilu is a practical philosopher in the hospital. If he has lost a limb he is thankful for the one that is left to him. If he is badly wounded he is glad it is not worse.

Someone has worked out in words the philosophy of the French soldier or the "Poilus' Litany" as follows:

"When I am mobilized, I shall either be kept in the rear or sent to the front. If I remain in the rear there is nothing to worry about. If I am sent to the front one of two things can happen. I shall either be sent to a post of no danger or to a dangerous position. If I am sent to a post of danger, one of two things can happen. I shall either be wounded or I shall not be wounded. If I am not wounded, there is nothing to worry about. If I am wounded, I shall either be slightly or severely wounded. If I am slightly wounded, there is nothing to worry about. If I am severely wounded, one of two things can happen. I shall either get well, in which case there is nothing to worry about, or I shall die, and then I can't worry."

Chapter XVI.

Fragments.

One day in the spring of 1916 as we were going into the dining room of the Hôtel du Grand Cerf at Senlis, we passed a French general who was leaving the room followed by several officers. The general was a medium-sized man with a grayish moustache. His strong but kindly face was marked with lines of care. A Belgian in our party exclaimed, "That is General Foch!" so we rushed to the window to have another look at him as he entered his limousine and succeeded in getting a snapshot.

Before the war Foch was well known as a professor in the military school at St. Cyr and his writings are standard works on military subjects. As Joffre's right-hand man he is recognized as the greatest strategist of the French Army. At the battle of the Marne General Foch commanded the Ninth army, and it was at the marshes of St. Gond that he executed his famous maneuver and sent his celebrated message: "My left is broken, my right is routed, therefore I will attack with the center."

We came very near having the distinguished general for a patient at one time. A hurry call was sent for an ambulance to go to an accident on the road not far from Meaux. When our ambulance arrived there they found a fine Rolls-Royce car badly damaged by a collision with a stout elm tree. The passengers were no less than the famous General Foch and his son-in-law. They were both injured but, as it turned out, not seriously. Traveling along the narrow road lined with trees, at a rapid rate, it had been a question of going into a tree or smashing into a peasant's cart containing some women and children, and the chauffeur chose the former. It was a narrow escape for the general and his loss from such an accident would have been most untimely. We offered him the best our hospital afforded but he preferred to go to the hospital at Meaux, where, on account of it being a military center, he would have superior telegraphic and telephonic communication. Our ambulance carried him to Meaux as he wished and returned to the hospital where everyone was disappointed that it did not bring back the distinguished patient.

The next day one of our nurses was at Meaux visiting a patient in the hospital and had the good fortune to see General Joffre and President Poincaré when they came to visit General Foch.

They say that Foch is the master mind of strategy of all France. He is very highly esteemed but for no one have the people the affection that they have for Joffre. Rarely has any man commanded the universal love and admiration of an entire people as does "Papa" Joffre.

Someone brought a copy of Miss Aldrich's book, "A Hilltop on the Marne," to the ambulance and we learned, on consulting the map, that her little village of Huiry was within a few miles of us. One day we started out to find it but, on arriving at the Marne, we could not cross the river as the bridge had been blown up before the battle and had not yet been repaired. Another day we had better success by crossing the Marne higher up, where we found a bridge that had been put in shape again. By following an automobile map, we traced our way along the country roads until we reached the charming village on the hilltop. There was no need of enquiring for Miss Aldrich's home as it stood before us just as she described it with its "six gables, jumble of roofs and chimneys." The "small garden" was there "separated from the road by an old, gnarled hedge of hazel." Apparently we were first mistaken for Cook's tourists for which breed Miss Aldrich has a holy horror and shudders at the thought that four hundred have already registered to visit her nest after the war. When we properly identified ourselves we received a cordial American welcome. The view from her terrace was all that she claimed for it, "a panorama rarely seen equaled," and it is described so much better in her book than I could write about it that no description shall be attempted. With field glasses we could plainly see the villages scattered over the Marne valley and could see the battlements of Juilly partly hidden in a hollow.

From the gifted authoress' vivid description we felt that we ourselves had stood there as she did when the cannon roared, the air was thick with smoke of shells and burning villages and the fading cannon shot told her that the foe was in retreat. Amélie, Aberlard and the donkey were all there, just as described. We saw the wood where the Uhlans had hidden and the road where the Irish scout had fallen off his bicycle when the effects of the large drink of eau de vie de prunes had come upon him.

Late one winter's night at the end of January, 1916, we were aroused by a peculiar roaring sound in the sky which came from the direction of Paris and faded away in the distance towards the front. Along with it we recognized the familiar sounds of aeroplanes and could hear the reports of cannon towards Paris. The next day we learned that Paris had suffered a Zeppelin raid and that these monsters must have passed over our village on their return. A few houses demolished, huge holes in the pavements, a score or so of men, women and children killed in their beds, the French people more determined than ever — such were the results of the raid. What a stupid method of warfare! Not one stroke of military value accomplished and the raids in England are the best means of stimulating recruiting.

One day we were surprised to see a British aviator walk into the ambulance and enquire if there was anyone here who could speak English. As he had run short of gasolene and oil, he had descended in a nearby field and left the aeroplane in charge of his comrade while he started out in quest of these necessities. He seemed somewhat surprised to find American men and women in the war zone but concealed his surprise in accordance with the tenets of English good form. He did not volunteer to tell us where he had come from or where he was going and we did not think it was polite to ask him. He said, however, that as he was descending he was glad to find that French peasants with their rods for driving oxen did not turn out to be Uhlans with lances.

After supplying his lack of gasolene and oil and taking a hasty lunch, he departed in a hurry, not forgetting his comrade, as his pockets were well filled with bread and cheese.

A few days later came a polite letter from Paris thanking us for our hospitality, so we at least found out his destination.

On Washington's Birthday I attended the banquet of the American Club as a guest of Mr. Benét, president of the club. The dinner was an excellent one, given in the large banquet room of the Hotel Palais d'Orsay and was attended by about two hundred guests.

The finest thing of the evening was the speech of Henri Bergson, the famous French philosopher. He gave an analysis of Washington's character and achievements that was a masterpiece. He spoke in simple language, in clear, beautiful French so that I hardly missed a word. Several times he quoted from Washington's farewell address and from other writings, quoting from memory and using perfect English. There were

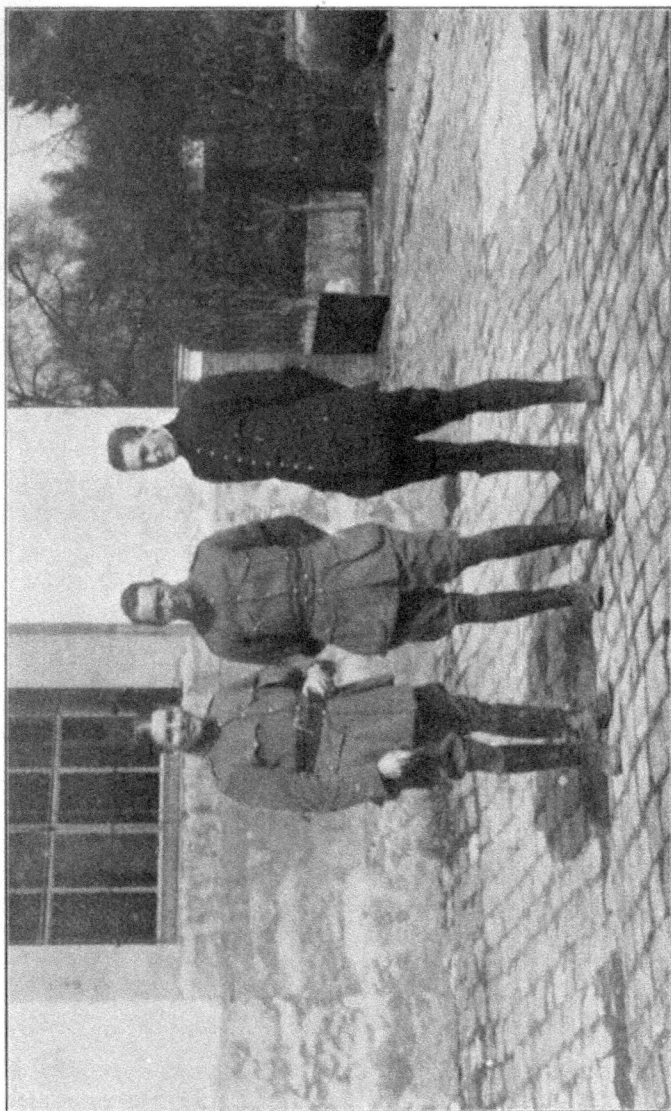

The American Aviators Prince, McConnell and Rockwell

other speeches in English and French (one by Denys Cochin, Minister of State) but none to compare with Bergson's. To end the evening's pleasure an American read a long, dry speech, which almost spoiled the whole evening.

Some of my letters home were published in the local newspapers. Among other incidents I related that a field hospital was bombed by German aviators and this was kept up on succeeding days, even when the location of the hospital was changed. The publication of this incident brought forth a protest from a local German that it could not be true and a request for further investigation. A round robin published by five American war correspondents, Bennet, McCutchen, Cobb, Hansen and Lewis, about alleged German cruelties in Belgium was adduced as an argument that such accusations were without any foundation. I refused to enter into a controversy at 8000 miles distance and replied that time and history would decide whether atrocities had been committed or not. The inadequacy of a "round robin" of any war correspondents on the German side is very evident, as any acquaintance with the methods of the German staff shows that what the correspondents are allowed to observe is carefully attended to in the German system. The war correspondents on the German side are so carefully chaperoned that they see only what the staff wants them to see. The overwhelming evidence from Belgium and Northern France as to burning, pillaging, rapine and murder of innocent civilians as part of Germany's system of frightfulness will be presented and proven to the world in a way that can not be explained away by German subtlety and trickiness.

Richard Norton of Boston in charge of the American Volunteer Motor-Ambulance Corps attached to one of the divisions of the French armies, made an interesting point in one of his letters concerning Germany's preparedness in the use of poisonous gas. After quoting the Bulletin of Information, distributed to the troops on October 1st, 1915, which states the numbers of prisoners and cannons captured in the Champagne offensive, he says :

"In this notice no mention is made of some very interesting gas machines that were taken. They were of two sorts, one for the production of gas, the other to counteract its effects. The latter were rather elaborate and heavy but very effective instruments consisting of two main parts; one to slip over the head, protecting the eyes and clipping the nose, the other an arrangement of bags and bottles containing oxygen, which the wearer inhaled through a tube held in the mouth. There were several forms of these apparatus, but the most interesting point to note about them is that one had stamped upon it the words: 'Type of 1914—developed from type of 1912, developed from type of 1908,' thus showing that seven years ago the Germans had decided to fight with gas."

One cannot but be impressed with the devotion and spirit of sacrifice of the French people. The cry "Liberty, Equality and Fraternity," a hundred years or so ago made the poorly paid and equipped armies of the French revolution irresistible. In 1870 the same spirit was there but France was poorly led and the poilu never had a chance.

France has made large sacrifices and is willing to make more. "The Germans must be driven out and Prussianism must be overthrown, else our children and grandchil-

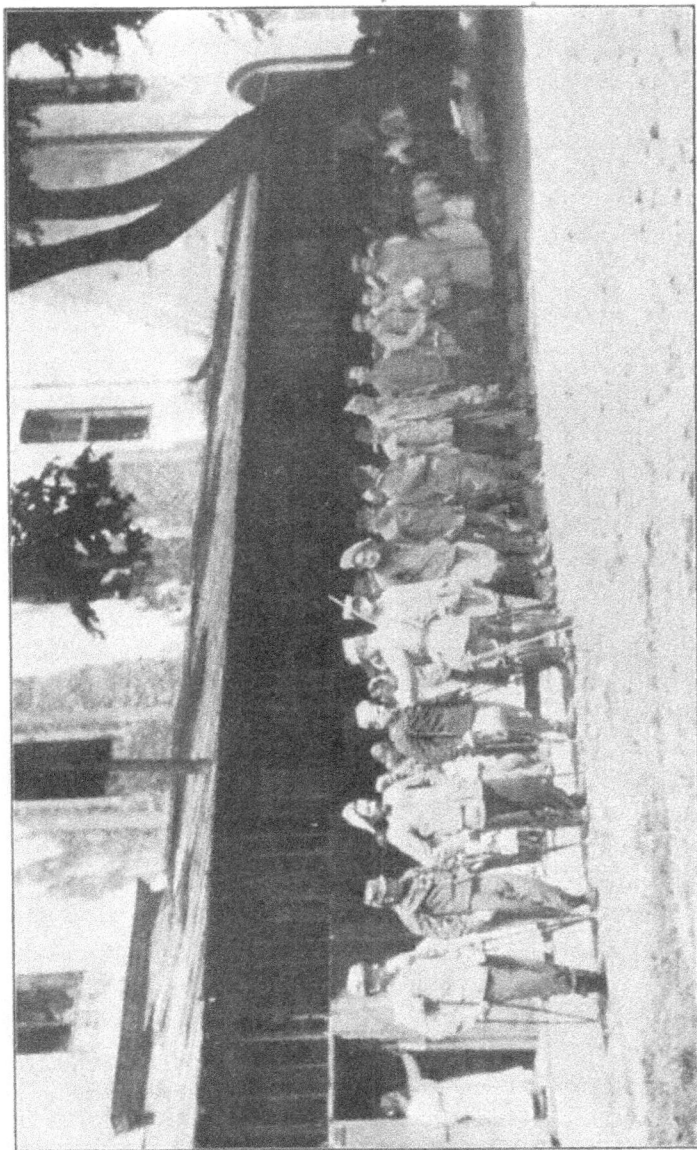

Decoration of sixteen heroes from Verdun—(One man on a stretcher.)

dren will be called on to defend France again. Better is it to make further sacrifices jusqu'au bout, for the sake of our children and their children."

The world knows of the steadfastness and bravery of the poilu, but not enough of the women of France. It is safe to say that France could not have held out had it not been for the women. A large number of shells fired at the invaders of their country are made by women's hands. White-haired grandmothers are working in the Red Cross. In the country it is a common sight to see women gathering in the crops. Children, too, of tender years are out in the fields in the cold rain, tending sheep, driving carts and helping with the harvest. It is not only in the way of replacing the men at productive tasks that the French women are so magnificent but it is their spirit which is so much to be admired. Women who have lost husbands, or sons, or brothers, are fulfilling their daily tasks with smiling faces, inspiring with their brave spirit the soldier in the trenches.

Chapter XVII.

Soldiers' Stories

The colonel was in command of a body of the famous Colonial troops in the offensive. They left the firing line at 9:15 on the morning of September 25th and charged for the German trenches under heavy shell fire. The colonel felt himself hit several times, but suffered no pain and was not disabled. The German trench was reached and there was some fierce hand to hand fighting. Right into a crowd of his men a bomb was thrown and lay smoking on the floor of the trench. There was not a moment to lose. The colonel seized the bomb and threw it back towards the Germans. As he hurled it away, it exploded and his hand was blown to pieces. He then became conscious of great pain and was evacuated to the rear. When he reached our hospital we found him suffering from twelve wounds. After months of hospital treatment necessary for his recovery, he again reported for duty with request for active service.

One day during his convalescence we went for a drive and, as we rested on a hill which commanded a superb view of the fertile plain, dotted with groves of trees and little villages, the colonel looked out and exclaimed, "Well, this is a land worth fighting for!"

One of our blessés from Verdun was a ruddy-faced, stalwart sergeant. When I examined his scalp wound he showed me his steel helmet with a bullet hole in it and told this story:

"In one of the furious attacks at Verdun we were charging the Germans with the bayonet. Directly in front of me on a little mound was a tall Prussian officer with a great plume in his helmet. He had a revolver in his hand and as I charged towards him, he pointed it at different parts of me, first at my stomach, then at my chest. I expected any moment to receive the ball.

Finally when I was barely two metres away he fired at my head. I felt a blow on my head and my casque was knocked off."

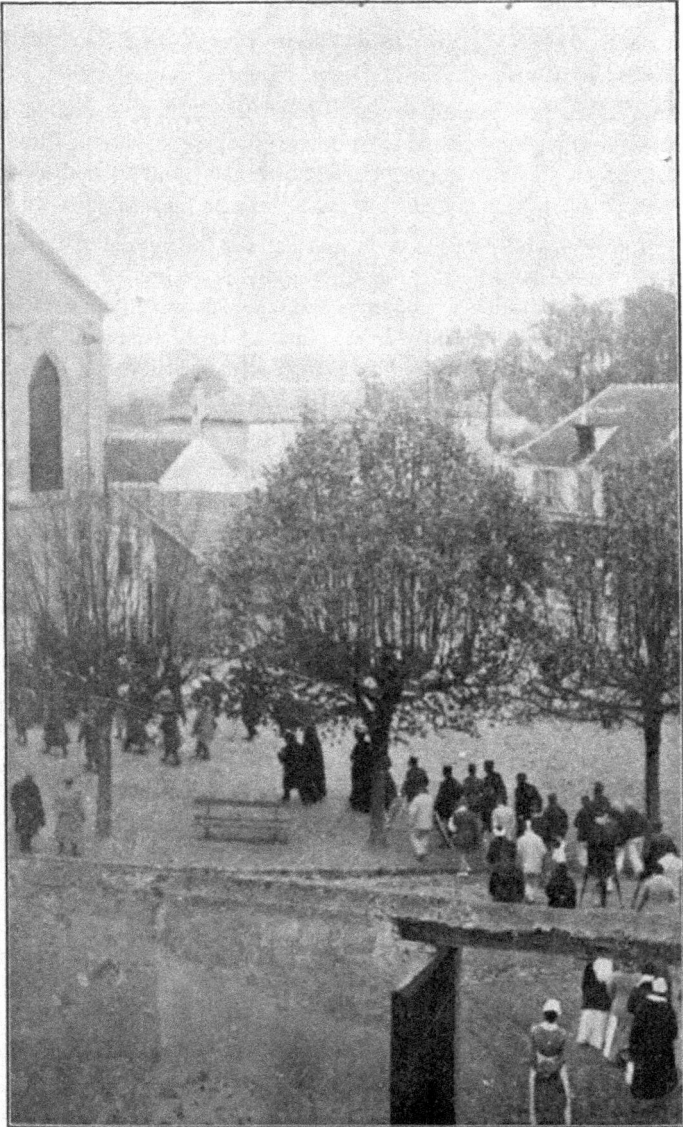

A funeral procession going from the hospital to the village church.

He then paused, so I asked, "And what happened then ?"

He replied, "Well, I kept right on running."

"What happened next?" I asked.

"I took these field glasses off from around his neck and I' am glad to give them to you as a souvenir of Verdun."

A well-known American manufacturer of artificial legs established a branch office in Paris. Thanks to the generosity of friends every amputé goes out of Juilly hospital walking on two feet. The gift of an artificial leg costing 500 francs is a very practical form of charity as it enables a man in many cases to resume his trade and support his family.

A soldier reformé, whose leg has been amputated at the middle of the thigh, comes out from Paris to take the necessary measurements and attend to the fittings. He walks with scarcely a limp and may be said to be a walking advertisement for his firm. Our artificial leg measurer was wounded in the battle of the Marne, near Barcy, which is only a few miles from Juilly. He related his story to us as follows:

"Before the war I was a grocer. I was mobilized at the onset and sent into active service. I went through all the horrors and hardships of the retreat from the Belgian frontier. At times we marched along, sound asleep, and our comrades fell in the road from exhaustion. We didn't know what was going to happen to us. We were at the limit of our endurance. When the order came that we were to make a stand and die rather than give way further, it was welcomely received. Our regiment was soon engaged with the Boches and we went at them with determination in our hearts and the consciousness that we were driving them back from our women and children.

"The second day of the battle we were fighting in the open fields at close quarters late in the afternoon. I was on one knee firing at the Germans, when a rifle ball struck me near the knee and tore up my thigh. I fell over, my comrades passed on and I lay out in the field in a half-conscious condition. I was aroused several hours later by the sound of voices, speaking German. It was dark and in the distance flashes of cannon lit up the night. I was carried by the Germans to the town of Vareddes, near by, where I was dumped on the floor of the Mairie along with many other wounded. Here I lay for three days on the stone floor with some water and a few pieces of bread to sustain me. I saw limbs cut off without anaesthetics. The shrieks of the sufferers were terrible. The odor of my leg warned me that I was in a bad way. Suddenly, on the fourth day, the Germans departed, driven out by the French.

"I was one of six wounded placed in a large truck and sent to Paris. Three of us arrived there alive. We were taken to a hospital. I was delirious but conscious enough to hear the doctor say there was no use in amputating my leg. It was too late. I roused up and begged the doctor to amputate and give me the chance. He agreed. I do not remember much what happened during the next few weeks but I gradually recovered and in three months was out of the hospital. One day, limping along on my crutches, I saw a sign 'American Artificial Legs.' I entered the shop and made arrangements to obtain one. I became interested in the construction and fitting of the leg and delighted when I found I could use it so readily. On account of my speaking some English the

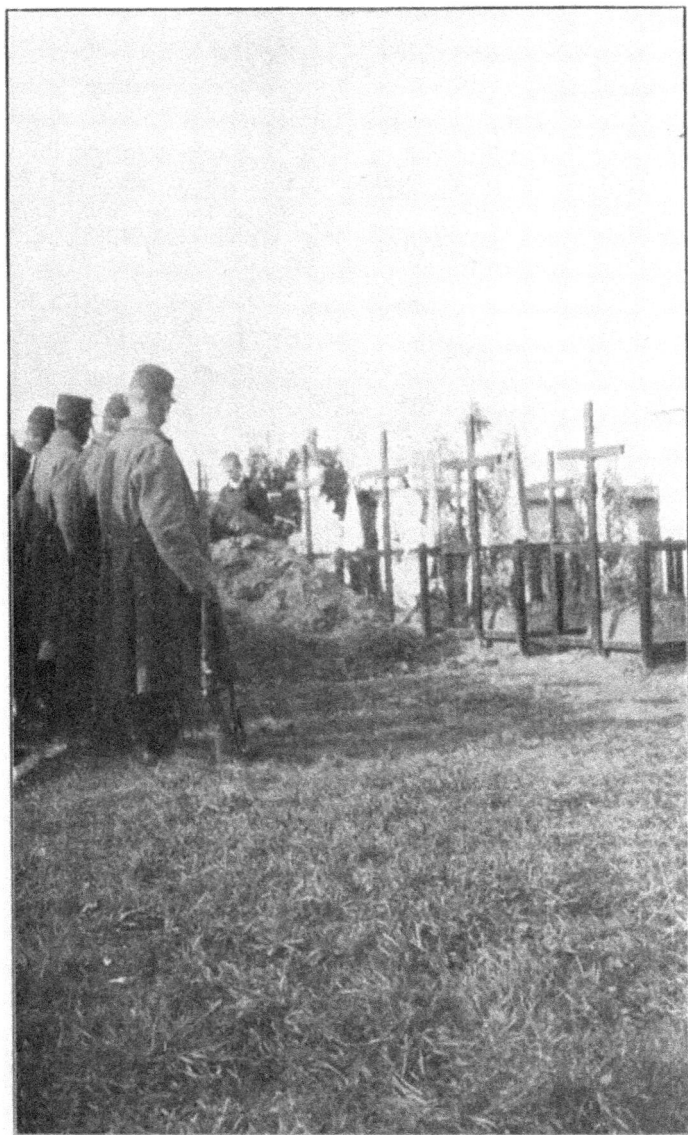

A soldier's burial.

manager offered me a position and so now I have changed from a grocer into an artificial leg artisan and I have fitted several hundred legs and know there will be many more."

A School Teacher's Story.

A reservist of the active army, I was called the second day of mobilization to join my regiment. The 5th of August, 1914, we departed for the eastern front. My regiment formed at this time the part of the second army in command of General Dubail. Our duty was to advance into Lorraine by Sarrebourg. The advance commenced from the 8th of August and on the 14th I found myself for the first time in contact with Bavarian infantry. It is not easy to give an exact idea of my first impressions of combat. It rests in my mind like a dream bordering on a nightmare. The sharp whistling of the bullets, the overwhelming roar of the cannonade, the cries of the wounded, the death rattle, the irresistible, "En avant, à la baïonnette," then the dead bodies, the wounded begging to be carried off the field, the broken guns and equipment scattered here and there, furnish a picture never to be forgotten and impossible to describe in words. I have seen other combats since, attacks and hand to hand fighting, but they have never left the impression on me like the first encounter.

The Bavarians had to retreat. Proud of our first success we marched ahead and on the 15th of August we crossed the frontier singing the "Marseillaise," with our flag unfurled at the head of the regiment. The frontier boundary post was torn up with general enthusiasm and cries of "Vivent l'Alsace et Lorraine." Alas! our joy was a passing one. On the 16th we arrived in sight of Sarrebourg. Saluted by a hail of artillery we advanced now very slowly, marching at. wide intervals, while about us the "Marmites" fell with a deafening noise, marking their passage by large holes, veritable tombs dug by infernal shovels. They were real tombs, because the unhappy victims sleep now their last sleep in these shell holes. Some troops penetrated to Sarrebourg where they were feted by the inhabitants, or at least by those who had remained French. Flowers, cigars, cakes and wines were for them gifts of welcome. These bodies of troops were forced to stop at the exit of the city as the enemy artillery cut them down. For my part I was busy with my section in a field of oats digging individual "abris" which would protect us somewhat against the balls. These shelters were our dining rooms, lounging and bed rooms. Smoking became a delicate operation, a wise art. As to exposing oneself, it was not to be thought of. The six biscuits and the can of meat called "monkey-meat" by the soldiers, were all we had to eat for these two days. During the night of August 18th we were able to retire to a small village several kilometres from Sarrebourg, where we had the pleasure of sleeping three long hours on fresh piles of hay. At 2 o'clock in the morning the arrival of shells in the village announced itself by a tremendous crashing of roofs. It was necessary to retreat and now the advance guard had to pass through Sarrebourg again. The German element exultingly showed their satisfaction of seeing the flight of the red pantaloons by firing on them from the windows with rifles and revolvers. The enemy troops pursued our advance guard and inflicted considerable loss on them. Unfortunately the fight was too unequal. We were overwhelmed by the shells which, minute by minute, followed each other in groups of six. We lacked artillery to cause similar losses in the ranks of the enemy. Retreat commenced at nightfall. What a turmoil! Pursued, confused, we fled on all sides, not knowing where to go. We had to tramp across the fields in the dark night over bad and unknown roads. Miles succeeded miles. At each instant one fell over exhausted soldiers sleeping in the fields or along the sides of the road. These we roused or dragged along to abandon again to their fatigue some distance beyond. Others trailed behind too far where, unhappy thought, they were taken prisoners by the Boches. How many thus fell into the hands of the Germans! The 21st of August we again crossed the frontier, but this time it was to return into France. The frontier post was there, lying in the river bed. It seemed to reproach us now in waiting for the Germans to replace it, to carry it further back perhaps. We will take it again, we will carry back the frontier post to the other side of the Rhine even if it takes our last man!

After several unsuccessful attempts to take the offensive we arrived near the forts of Epinal. Our lines were reorganized and we prepared to undertake a vigorous offensive. On the 28th we drove the Germans out of a nearby village while the chasseurs alpins, who had come to our aid, captured another village in a furious bayonet charge. There I saw, after this combat, one of our soldiers and a German infantryman standing upright against a wall each one of them transfixed with a bayonet and still holding their muskets in spite of death which had done its work some time before.

We now advanced rapidly. The Germans, not being supported by their heavy artillery, were incapable of withstanding our offensive. We passed through villages bombarded and burned all in ruins, not a house standing. Most of them were a pile of ruins. From this débris there was already a nauseating odor of decaying animals, which had not been able to get away; of human beings too, perhaps under those ruins. Early in September we reached the banks of the Meurthe. Tomorrow we shall again be at the frontier. Alas! No! We have to make a detour and go to support at St. Mihiel the shock of the Crown Prince's army, which is resolutely advancing on this side, while to the north our troops are drawing quickly back before the German assault. It has since been said that St. Mihiel and Nancy formed the pivot of the maneuver. It was this pivot it was necessary to defend. Severe fighting ensued at le Grand Couronné, near Nancy. Towards St. Mihiel, which was defended by forts, there were only skirmishes. The enemy attacked the forts. They launched three unsuccessful attacks against the fort of Troyon.

We were called to aid the army at the Aisne after they had driven back the Germans at the battle of the Marne. We arrived at St. Menehould, then we marched to the Camp of Châlons but after one stage we returned. The enemy had succeeded in capturing the fort of Troyon. We had to return to where we were three days before and attack the Germans occupying the village of Apremont.

In the early days of October we occupied the redoubts of the fort of Lionville. There for eight days we had to submit to a most violent bombardment. An entire section of my company with the captain were engulfed in one of the redoubts. It was impossible to rescue them. After such a bombardment the enemy attacked, always in compact masses according to their custom. Their losses were enormous. Mowed down by our machine guns, the heaps of corpses preserved very clearly the formation of columns by fours. French and Germans were on the watch at 50 meters from each other. It was impossible to bury the dead and, from time to time, shells from both sides struck these corpses and blew them into pieces. Cruel profanation.

After a month there we retired about two kilometers in the rear for a rest. There I was wounded in the right shoulder by a piece of shell. I was far from expecting such an occurrence at this time, when I thought I was in safety. I was evacuated and after thirty hours of cruel suffering on the train I reached the hospital where I was taken care of until I reported at my dépôt. I was soon again at the front. Now it was the war of the trenches, a warfare not interesting. I remained there five months without noting a single event really interesting. I saw only one casque à pointe, which one was that of a prisoner. From time to time an insignificant bombardment, the periodical flooding of the trenches with water, the digging that went on, the games of cards at the bottom of a hole, the silence of the night disturbed occasionally by a rifle shot fired by a sentinel who, struggling against the desire for sleep, tries to keep himself awake by shooting. Voilà la guerre en tranchées. Twenty days in the trenches, twenty days of repose.

The first of August, after violent pain, my wound of last year broke open and discharged. I was evacuated to Compiègne and from there to Juilly. At the American Hospital they extracted the piece of shell which for nine months was for me a very troublesome guest. Now I am almost well.

I would fear to offend the modesty of the doctors and nurses if I set forth their merits. Let me simply say that I have found among the Americans who have left their land to come to France to care for their wounded brothers, a devotion, vigilant attention and constant care which makes me admire them and in them admire the great nation, sister of France beyond the Atlantic, the United States of America.

In thanking them all from the bottom of my heart, I terminate my little story.

We cared for one soldier of the Foreign Legion. He was an architect living in Chicago, an American of French descent. There was nothing warlike in his nature but he could not withstand the call of the blood when France was invaded.

A FOREIGN LEGION SOLDIER'S STORY.

I left my home in Chicago in the middle of September, 1914, and boarded the French liner "Rochambeau" at New York. After an uneventful trip of nine days I landed at Havre, where I enlisted in the Foreign Legion.

The Foreign Legion now serving in the war against Germany has little in common with the two world famous regiments stationed in Algeria. While most of our officers were drawn from those regiments only two battalions were sent out from Africa to "encadrer" the foreign volunteers. The remainder were either kept in Algeria and Morocco or sent to the Dardanelles or to some distant colony like Indo-China.

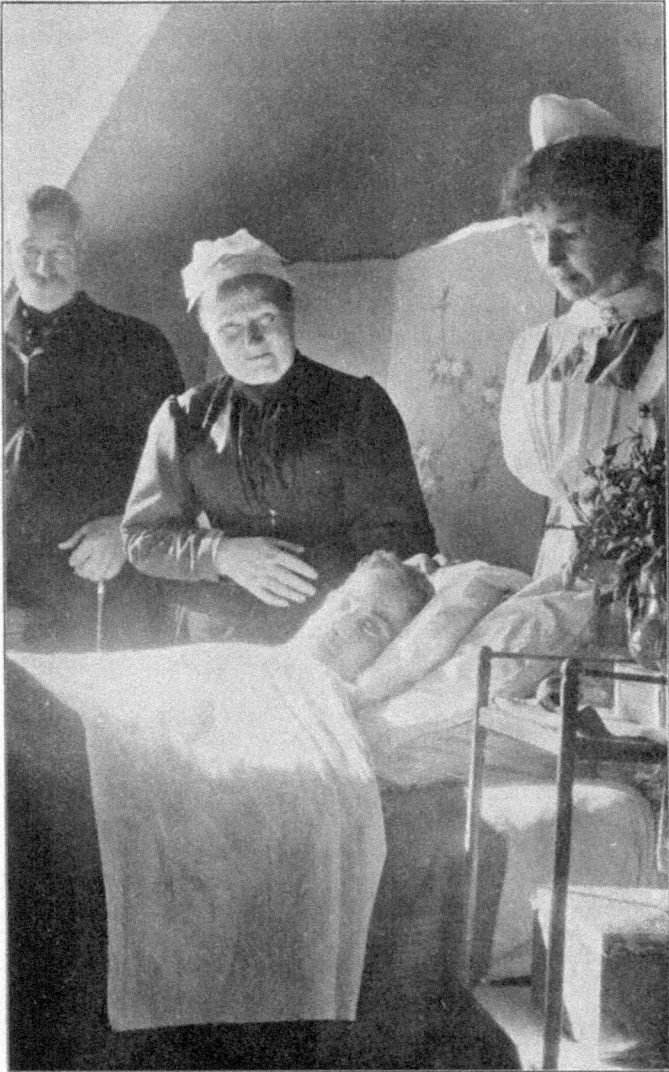

French peasants at the bedside of their wounded son.

In order to train the foreign volunteers six dépôts were provided. The second regiment had three dépôts— Toulouse, Orleans and Blois. I was sent to Toulouse where battalion C was being organized and two days after my arrival I witnessed the departure of that battalion for the front. A very picturesque sight it was to see them go, all brave hearts, ready to sacrifice themselves for the cause of France. Each of them was flying on his knapsack the colors of his respective country. Uncle Sam was represented by a good sprinkling of the Stars and Stripes lost amidst a greater number of Russian, English, Belgian and other flags.

After a two months' hard drilling, the dépôt was transferred to Orleans and I stayed there until January 25, 1915. I was then ordered to the front with a reinforcement 200 strong.

Our regiment with four battalions occupied a front about two miles long before the plateau of Craonne and the ruined city of that name, where the Germans are so strongly fortified that its capture would cost at least 50,000 men.

I soon got acquainted with the routine of the service. Six days trenches, six days rest. The part of our sector occupied by our company was about 1000 yards from the Germans and was therefore a quiet one. It would have been even more so, had it not been for the artillery of the Germans which daily showered on us fire and steel. No event of any importance occurred during my four months' stay there except the trial by court-martial of nine Russians who refused to go to the trenches. Found guilty, they were executed the next day at dawn.

There I came to know the real "Légionnaire" by which I mean the one from Africa. The following verses which I plagiarize from the comic opera "Les Mousquetaires au Couvent" quite well typifies them. I only substitute the word "Légionnaire" for "Mousquetaire:"

Pour être un brave Légionnaire
Il faut avoir l'esprit joyeux
Grand air et léger caractère
Aimer les femmes, boire encore mieux.
But good fellows after all and ready to help when sober.

We left Craonne in May and were sent to Sillery, a very bad place, where the battalion lost 150 men in one week. We were then shifted over to a place near Rheims and in July were sent to rest in the neighborhood of Belfort.

President Poincaré and General Joffre came to review us and we were presented with a flag which was well earned by ten months of warfare.

After a short time in Alsace, where I got a sight of the famous Hartmanswillerskopf of which so much has been written, we were ordered to Champagne with the whole Moroccan division, of which we were a part, and on the 25th of September took an active part in the general offensive.

On the 26th while entrenched on the plain in front of the "Ferme Navarin" as reserve of the 6th Army Corps, I volunteered in the midst of bursting shells to go and get some water for my squad. On my return I was struck by a shell which fractured my femur, missing the femoral artery by only a hair. Carried away from the field of battle to Souain I spent the night on a stretcher suffering with a terrible fever while the rain poured down. The next day the motor ambulance took me to Châlons and from there I was sent to the ambulance at Juilly where I found myself again in America. Thanks to the good care which I received my wounds soon healed up and the bone united so that I will be able to walk as well as ever.

To the end of the offensive the Legion, faithful to its glorious past, distinguished itself but was almost wiped out. The original number has very much dwindled and only one regiment is left under the name of Régiment de marche de la Légion Etrangère but it is as eager to fight and die for the cause of Right and Justice as it was on the first day of the war.

One of our blessés was a little rag picker. He was always smiling, so someone named him "Sunny Jim" and the name clung to him. As his comrades adopted the name the little poilu became proud of it and signed himself your grateful "Sanidaime." A German bullet had gone through his temple cutting the optic nerve of one eye but "Sunny Jim" was happy that he had one good eye.

After a few days our little poilu told us about his experiences in the Champagne offensives.

Sunny Jim's Story.

"At three o'clock the morning of September 25th, we left our camp for the 'tranchées de départ.' At five o'clock we arrived at our destination. There was a terrific bombardment going on. We filled our musettes with grenades. The news soon circulated in the trench that we would attack at a quarter past nine. The time passed as we sat quietly on the floor of the trench waiting for the opportunity to measure ourselves with the cursed Boches. At nine o'clock we stood ready. At nine ten we fixed bayonets. Suddenly a short order spread down the line. We sprang over the edge and crossed the barbed wire. As far as we could see on each side of us were our comrades running forward. This gave us courage. We arrived at the first line. There was not a live German there, only dead ones. Our artillery fire had destroyed the trench and we could see arms and legs sticking out of the earth. Some of our soldiers began to fall but we kept on and passed the second and third trenches which were as badly battered as the first. Then out in the open, bullets began to arrive in great numbers, also shells, but we kept on. Suddenly we came across a strong force of the enemy. Now it was time to know how to use the bayonet. We threw ourselves on them and the combat was on, a terrible mêlée. Steel met steel, and steel was driven into flesh until the Germans gave way and retreated. But we did not give them time to get. away. Just as we had advanced about a hundred metres a ball struck me in the head and laid me out senseless. I fell into the ditch along the roadside. I lay there twenty-four hours regaining consciousness several times only to faint away again. Finally during the night I came to myself. I was tortured by thirst. I had two bidons of water with me but I was too weak to raise myself. The next day stretcher bearers passed by and saw us. I was not alone, as a

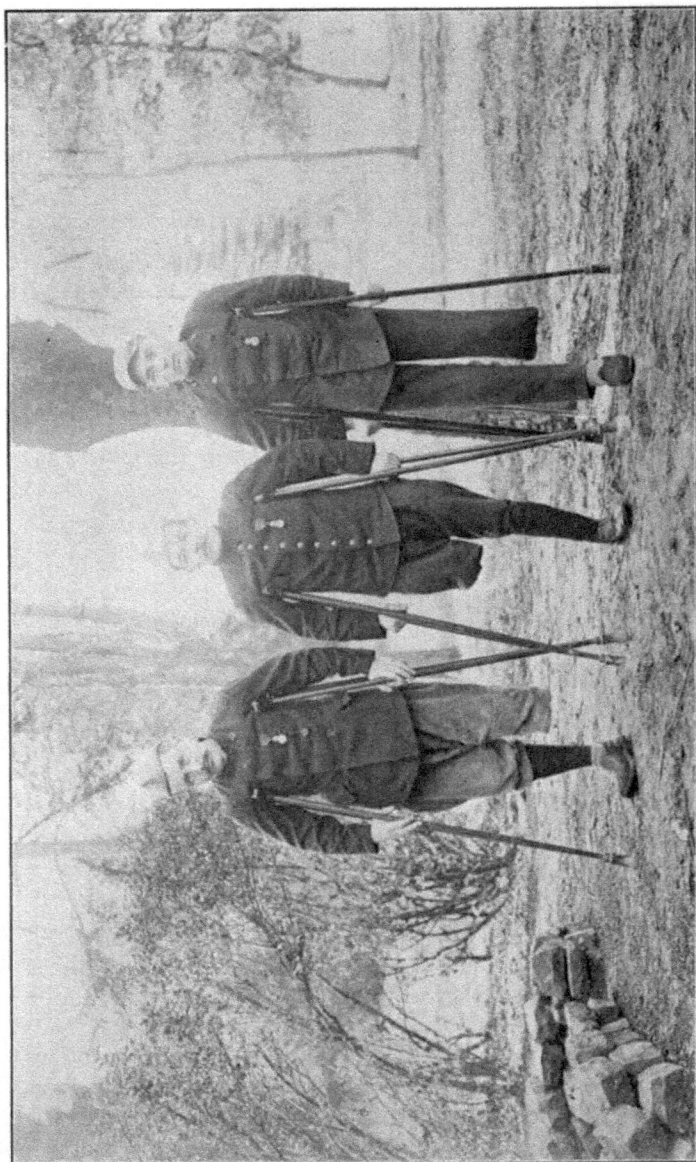

Before

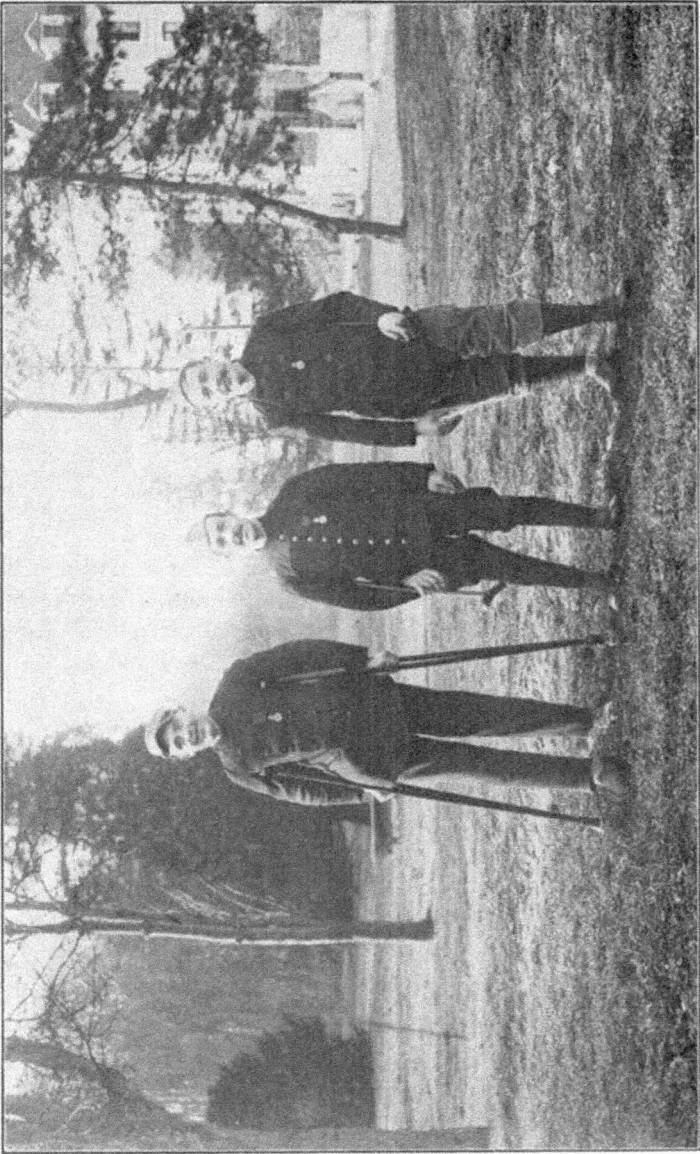

After

dead comrade lay alongside of me. They looked at us but thinking us both dead they were about to go on when I collected my forces sufficiently to cry out for something to drink. They then picked me up and carried me to Souain where I received the first dressing. From there I was taken to Châlons and after three days I was sent to Juilly. It will be with regret that I will quit this hospital for which I shall always have a pleasant and ineffaceable memory."

The Chasseur's Story.

I was mobilized the second of August, 1914. As soon as I arrived at my dépôt, we were sent to join the active forces in Belgium. We crossed the Belgian frontier on August 12th, and continued to Charleroi where the little Belgian soldiers fought like lions against the Boches but unfortunately we arrived too late and the retreat commenced.

The retreat was in good order. At one time we were the advance guard, clearing the road in order to avoid ambuscades, at other times we were the rear guard, protecting the retreat of our brothers in arms.

The first serious combat that I took part in was at Moy, a village between la Fère and St. Quentin. From seven in the morning to six at night we held the Germans, although we were inferior in number. Finally overwhelmed by numbers we had to retreat again in the direction of la Fère. We marched two days and two nights without halting and crossed the forest of Nouvion, which was full of Boche ambuscades. At the exit of this forest a detachment of English troops joined with us and on September 2nd the Paris autobuses picked us up and transported us to Nanteuil le Haudoin.

On September 6th we received the order of the commander in chief calling on us to hold our ground and to die rather than give way. The combat commenced on the sixth, about seven o'clock in the morning—a terrible struggle for three days and nights, when on the ninth of September the Boches began to waver in their resistance. That was a good augury for us and we redoubled our efforts, which brought about the retreat of the Germans. The pursuit commenced and continued to Château Thierry. There we had a rest of twenty-four hours and there we had the pleasure of cleaning up at least two hundred Germans whom we found in the cellars dead drunk on champagne, their favorite drink.

We were then carried by taxi-cabs to a village near Soissons, where we did not have much trouble in driving out the enemy, as they were on the run. In spite of that many corpses were strewn over the ground.

The German retreat continued to Berry an Bac, where I was wounded in the right shoulder by two bullets from a machine gun. I lay on the ground under fire of the enemy's artillery until night fall, when I reached a village, whence I was transported in a camion to the railroad station, where I met a number of other wounded. We piled into freight cars and reached the hospital at Dinan after thirty-six hours.

In six weeks I was back at the front. I rejoined my battalion on the heights of the Meuse. It was now the war of the trenches. The winter was not an unhappy one. There were not many attacks made or received. Each side saved his forces for the spring.

On the thirteenth of February the order was given to attack the crest of Eparges and we drove back the Boches to their last line of trenches, fighting with grenades, rifle buts and even with our fists. We were fortunate in not losing many men and our attack exceeded the expectations of our chiefs. Half of the crest was now in our possession. On the ninth of March we attacked again to take the rest. The attack was admirably carried out. Our artillery belched forth a storm of shells and the Boches drew back. After three days of fighting all the crest was in our hands save one position, the point X.

In spite of the enemy's counter attacks we remained masters of the crest although the enemy counter attacked seventeen times during the next twenty-four hours. Our losses in repulsing these counter attacks were heavy. In front of our trenches there was a veritable charnel house where our dead and the enemy's were piled up high.

On April 6th and 7th we again attacked the position X, and after a series of assaults the Boches were driven down the hill with heavy losses. Our commandant was killed by a ball in the forehead and shortly afterwards I was wounded by a piece of shell in the left shoulder. I did not see the end of the combat, as I was evacuated by an ambulance to the rear to Dugny, where I spent three weeks in the hospital.

On the first of August we were given a "repos" of forty-five days near Bar le Duc. How delicious it was, especially in August. Soldiers, civilians, women and children—everyone worked at reaping the harvest and housing the crops.

On September 10th we marched to the Champagne front and on the morning of the 25th we took part in the offensive. The terrain, swept by artillery fire, was prepared for us, the troops leaped over the parapet and we took the two first lines of the enemy's trenches, scarcely firing a shot. The artillery had well done its work.

The same day we attacked the second reserve, the last German lines. This terrible combat lasted all day, and in spite of heavy losses, we broke through their defenses and pursued them in the open. At dusk the rain began to fall and hindered our advance. We lay out in the mud all night, hastily fortifying the ground we had taken, and the rain never ceased to fall. What an anxious night amid the groans of the wounded and dying and we working in the rain with sad hearts.

Our patrols sent on in advance reported that the Boches were being reinforced and were fortifying themselves feverishly. At dawn we advanced again. Our captain was killed by a ball in the ear, the lieutenant was struck by a shell and the two sergeants, brave and good comrades, were killed on each side of me. As hardly any officers were left I was obliged to take command of our section as we were to attack the little fort of the bois Sabot.

It was no small undertaking to take this fortress, as it was defended by at least two hundred machine guns, which did not cease to sweep the ground. The soil was well covered with dead and wounded. For two hours we lay flat on the ground under a storm of bullets until our colonel gave the order to take this redoubt at any price. At this moment and as one man the two battalions rose and charged forward and after an hour or more of bayonet and grenade fighting we were masters of this fort. As booty we captured two hundred machine guns, two trench mortars, a pump for liquid fire and two apparatus for asphyxiating gas, besides a quantity of ammunition, rifles, grenades and other equipment.

Our battalion flag was cited in the Order of the Armies and proposed for the Legion of Honor.

The same night we were relieved by a battalion of Chasseurs, who continued the attack. During our return to the rear the Boches bombarded us with gas shells. I was wounded in the head by three pieces of shell, and I was almost asphyxiated by the gas that I inhaled. How long I lay on the ground I can't say. Two hours at least or perhaps less. When I came to myself I perceived a feeble light in the distance to which I directed myself, and had the good fortune to fall on to a "poste de secours," where my wounds were dressed. From there I was sent to Suippes, where I was placed on a sanitary train and sent to a hospital at La Rochelle.

After my wounds were healed, I reported at my dépôt whence I was sent to a section on the Pas-de-Calais, a rather quiet part of the line.

During a month's time we were on more or less good terms with the Bavarians opposite us and exchanged bread, chocolate, cigars and cigarettes until the Bavarians were relieved by a detachment of the Imperial Guard. The Prussians blew up seven mines under the trench where my company was stationed and buried all but eight of my company. Completely dazed, we joined ourselves to a small group of bombardiers of another company and we retook from the Boches 80 metres of trench by grenade fighting.

After being relieved from our position we had a short rest before we were ordered to Verdun.

For nine days in the first line the Boches attacked us twelve times with gas and liquid fire. These attacks with massed troops cost the Germans enormous losses. Our losses were heavy enough from the bombardment of cannon of all calibres, a bombardment never ceasing day and night. How many of my comrades lie there about our positions, still in death! It was a frightful sight to see, the dead heaped up in piles, dead horses, and pieces of caissons and cannon strewn around.

Our trenches were continually damaged by the explosion of "marmites" and for nine days and nights we had little rest. We were always engaged in watching the enemy day and night and in repairing the damage done to our trenches.

On the tenth day we were relieved from the first line to positions further back, where we were held in reserve, but there the "marmites" continually fell. I became an "agent de liaison" and carried orders from the Colonel of the Brigade. I carried on this duty for eight days, when I was wounded by a German shell in both legs, right hand and back. I was carried to the poste de secours, where I fainted. When I came to myself they lifted me into an American automobile having on its side a plate inscribed "don de la Société Hotchkiss." This car carried me to Revigny and from there I was evacuated to the American Ambulance of Juilly, where I recognized the driver who had carried me to Revigny.

I can only render homage to the doctors and nurses who have surrounded me with such good care during my stay here. Homage to America, our Sister Republic!

Chapter XVIII.

A Ttrip to the Front.

The land of the trenches always seemed a land of mystery to us. The booming of the cannon every day told us where the trenches lay, but a nearer acquaintance with the front was well nigh impossible for a non-combatant. Everyone in the ambulance had his or her place assigned and was not expected to step out of it. As time passed restrictions became more stringent. Each one of us was supplied with a "carnet d'étranger" which contained our photograph and signature and specific directions as to all movements in the war zone and this book had to be shown on going to Paris and returning by train. Our friends at Neuilly in the earlier months could visit us by procuring a pass following a week's application. Later this was shut down on and it was extremely difficult to obtain permission to go to Juilly. The authorities could not afford to have Americans or anyone else running around in the war zone.

In the early months of the war it was perhaps feasible for some of the American surgeons to visit the front, but in our time the matter was so difficult that it was not even attempted.

However, I reasoned that, having worked a year for the French wounded, I might be entitled to a trip to the front as a sort of recompense. Then, too, having come from such a far distance and being so near the front for so many months, the regret of missing this experience would always be a keen one. It would do no harm to try, so forthwith a letter was written to the Surgeon General at Headquarters requesting permission. A courteous reply was received in a few days enclosing a pass to Châlons, either by rail or auto. I chose the latter in order to see more of the country and to be more independent.

Early on a sunny morning in June I started with Fabrice, our Italian chauffeur, in the Médecin-Chef's limousine. We took the well-known road to Meaux along an edge of the Marne battlefield. Leaving Meaux with its picturesque old mills in the river and its venerable cathedral we passed through beautiful woods until we reached La Ferté Jouarre, where we crossed the Marne.

Near Napoleon's monument on the outskirts of Montmirail our trip nearly ended disastrously for we discovered that the car was on fire. The hot gases emerging from a hole in the muffler had ignited the oil-soaked wood work and one side of the car was blazing merrily. After tearing out the loose boards, waste, rags, extra tubes and inflammable material and hurling them out of the way, we tried in vain to beat out the fire with our overcoats. If it had not been for some water in a wheel rut near by, our trip would have ended then and there and our car would have been reduced to cinders and scrap iron. The kindly shade of an elm tree kept the water from drying up by the sun's rays. Our caps answered for fire buckets to get the fire under control, and a peasant with a bucket of water did the rest. just at that time a military car came along at a great rate of speed, its wheels grinding into the very rut which had been our salvation. Another remarkable thing was that along all the 125 kilometres that we did that day no other rut with water in it was seen. We thanked our lucky star that the fire had not reached the gasolene tank, crawled into Montmirail with a careful watch alongside and, after some delay, found a mechanic who made the necessary repairs.

From there on to Châlons the road ran straight as an arrow and smooth as a billiard table—the kind of road one reads about in novels but hardly expects to ever enjoy. Red poppies mingled with the blue of the corn flower, grew in profusion, and only needed the white shine of the road to complete the tricolor.

No other accident stopped us, but we were halted at every railroad crossing by Territorials who examined our pass in a critical manner.

Châlons is famous historically for the defeat of Attila, the Hun, by the Romans and Goths in 451 A. D. The town was full of bustle and excitement for it is a great army center. The principal hotel with the strange name of L'hôtel Haute Mère Dieu, was full of officers at lunch time, and I managed to find an inconspicuous place in the dining room. It was an interesting sight to watch the officers of different types, from stout, white-haired generals to young dapper lieutenants. I thought I was the only American for miles around until I ran into A. Piatt Andrew, Director of the Field Ambulance Service, who was taking Will Irwin and Arthur Gleason to write up an American Field Service section for the instruction of the American public.

According to my instructions, I presented my credentials at the Service de Santé, and was courteously received by General Bechard, and a fine limousine was placed at my disposal with a colonel of the medical service as my conductor.

The General mapped out a plan of a three days' visit to the hospitals of Châlons and field hospitals toward the front and then asked if there was anything more he could do for me. I replied that "I wanted very much to go to the trenches." "Ah," he said, "that is a military matter and you can only obtain permission from military headquarters." This advice was not encouraging but was enlightening. So for the present there was nothing to do but enjoy the many interesting things to see and reserve a trip to the trenches for the dernier coup.

As Châlons is an important military center there are a large number of hospitals there, admirably organized and equipped. Among the number of hospitals visited was one for mental cases—for brains unbalanced by the strain of war. There were a variety of types of mental aberration-manias, melancholics, delusions fixed and fleeting, mutism in different forms. It was sad indeed to see what war had done to these young minds, but with it all there was hope that time, rest and quiet would work an improvement. There was not the hopeless depression one feels on entering a ward of blind soldiers.

A book could be written on the different phases of mental disorders caused by this warfare. I shall merely relate the features of the curious case of a young artist. He was a well-dressed, trim young chap, and whenever he saw any button unbuttoned, he took it on himself to button it. He never spoke a word and apparently did not hear anything, as he paid no attention to noises or to anything that was said to him. For amusement he painted pretty little views of the hospital garden or fanciful scenes of meadows, streams and willow trees. All efforts to get him to write his name or initials on any of his paintings failed. Curious that a mind that could produce a painting faithful to nature, should lose its identity to the extent of being unable to claim the authorship.

East of Châlons towards the front at varying intervals about 12 miles back of the trenches are located a number of ambulances which we visited. These field hospitals are a series of low, wooden buildings located usually in some hollow and further hidden from hostile aviators by branches of trees placed on the roofs. Here the wounded are received directly by automobile from the Postes de Secours or dressing stations. There are also bathing establishments where a regiment can be cleaned up in a day. The soldiers get a hot shower bath and a hair cut and have their clothes fumigated.

Beautifying the field hospitals are well kept flower gardens. There are band stands for occasional concerts, and reading rooms and small theatres are provided for the poilus. Near the entrance to one of the buildings was a large hole made by a bomb dropped a few days ago by a hostile aviator. Close at hand is always the little cemetery with the graves close together marked by white crosses. One of the ambulances occupies an old farm, and its old stone buildings, stables and box-stalls have been converted into a well equipped institution.

Of special interest was an automobile field hospital. This was well equipped and so arranged that everything could be packed in trucks and moved to any desired location. Electricity was furnished by a dynamo run by a truck engine and the X-ray apparatus was similarly supplied.

All these sights were very interesting but the proximity to the trenches made me all the more anxious to visit them. I interviewed my conductor on the subject and asked him why I couldn't get permission to go. He said "Because we don't want a shell to come along and take your head off." He added that he had not been to the trenches himself as the work there is done by the younger men. I then asked him if he would go to the Quartier-General and ask permission for me. He politely told me he would introduce me, but would rather that I spoke for myself. To my complaint that I could hardly speak French well enough to address a general he smiled and said that I could make myself well understood. I then prepared my speech and rehearsed it to the colonel on our way to headquarters. When we arrived at General Gouraud's Etat Major we were formally saluted by the sentinel on duty as we entered the modest brick building. We received word that General Gouraud was absent but that his Chief of Staff would see us. An orderly, after a short wait, ushered us into a plainly furnished room, the walls covered with maps, where we were received by the Chief of Staff, an elderly, dignified man. After being introduced by the Colonel I made my speech and thanks to my preparation got through it quite well. The General listened seriously to what I had to say and then told me that he would present my request to the Commanding General, who alone could give the necessary permission. An answer would be sent me to the hotel. That night about half-past nine, as I was sitting in the hotel dining room chatting with some officers, a soldier entered and presented me with a letter by hand, as he was instructed. I almost hesitated to open the letter, feeling sure that my request would meet a polite refusal. However, much to my joy the letter said that Capt. —— would have the honor to call for me at half-past seven the next morning.

The next day was one of the most exciting of my life. The excitement started in at five o'clock in the morning when I was awakened by the noise of cannon rattling the window frames. I ran to the window and looked out and there, racing across the clear, blue sky, was a tiny black object. The cannon were firing at it and making the peculiar hollow sound they make when shooting in the air. The shells were exploding with their decisive little pop around the Taube and at once the rounded, white clouds appeared near the aeroplane. I counted twenty-seven of these rounded clouds, forming a track across the clear, blue heaven, but none of the shells hit the Taube, although they seemed to come very close to it. It was an interesting and spectacular sight. Three bombs were dropped by the German but did little damage. However, previous attempts had been more successful. On the main street near the hotel were the ruins of a house completely demolished by a bomb. Another bomb had dropped in the street in front of the cathedral and had broken some of the stained glass windows and peppered the walls of the adjacent buildings. Long before half past seven I was walking up and down before the hotel. Just at the hour a long, rakish, military car drove up and a trim officer jumped out and we introduced ourselves with the usual formalities.

In company with several officers we started off at a great rate of speed due North. One of the first things I noticed was a Winchester rifle strapped to the back of the front seat. On the outskirts of Châlons we were stopped by sentinels and our pass carefully scrutinized. Five miles from Châlons we came to the village of Lepine, completely burned by the Germans in their retreat after the battle of the Marne, with the exception of the remarkably beautiful church.

From there on a scene of great activity prevailed. We passed companies of troops coming back from the trenches—tired and dusty poilus. There were vehicles of most every description passing along the road—great ammunition camions, motor trucks laden with supplies, army wagons, cannon, armored cars, movable kitchens, water carts, motor cyclists and even a special motor truck for a carrier pigeon equipment. Along the road were well arranged water stations where the wants of man and beast could be supplied. From time to time we passed forges, where horses and mules were being shod and broken wagons and artillery carriages were being repaired. I wondered how the road stood all the traffic and was in such good condition until I saw several gangs of soldiers busily engaged in keeping it in repair. The little villages near the road were full of soldiers resting, washing their clothes, reading, talking and smoking. The activity of providing for a great army was everywhere apparent. There were great piles of hay along the roadside, stacks of timber ready for the trenches, barbed wire rolls heaped up in great piles, rows of shells, boxes of many kinds of stores. Away off in a corral was a herd of cattle which was to supply the army with fresh beef. Military cars passed us going at a great rate of speed and throwing up clouds of dust. Occasionally we met detachments of cavalry.

As we sped on our route over the thirty-five kilometres that separate Châlons from the front, we began to hear cannon boom in the distance ahead of us. A huge captive balloon, shaped like a sausage, could be seen miles away over the plateau. I knew it was huge, because although it was very high up, it looked enormous. I asked if it was French and was told that it was a German balloon over the German trenches but some distance back. This was my first sight of the German side and the reality of things began to be impressive. Off on the left towards Rheims three "saucissons" indicated to us where the French lines were. At the rapid rate of speed we travelled, we soon reached a little village sheltered behind a hill, where we dismounted from our automobile. Here we were received by the Major in charge and were equipped with steel helmets and masks. I asked if these things were necessary and was informed that there was no telling where a shell would burst and, as for the masks, the gas would travel five or six kilometres if the wind was favorable. There was some difficulty in finding a casque large enough to fit me. Finally after trying several, one was found which made a fair fit, but I found it heavy and uncomfortable. However, I was very glad to wear it. The gas mask was enclosed in a tin box and this I securely fastened to my belt. Thus equipped we started for Suippes, a short distance away. As we came in shell range and saw the freshly made shell-holes and heard the cannon's noise, now very loud, I must own to a feeling of fear, and I believe that the man who says he has no fear when he goes under fire for the first time is a liar. At the same time along with the fear there was a feeling of exhilaration and a desire to see it through.

We dashed through what was once the prosperous town of Suippes, now badly battered by shell fire and deserted. The only person to be seen on the long main street was a priest hurrying along on foot. He was clad in a black cassock and had a steel helmet on his head. We stopped on the outskirts of Suippes at a small château hidden in a grove of woods. Needless to say this was used as a hospital for badly wounded men, too badly damaged to stand further transportation. The cellar of the building was in readiness to be used in case the bombardment became dangerous. The Médecin-Chef received us cordially, and served champagne, tea and cakes in the garden. He said that an hour before two German shells had passed over the trees and fallen in the fields on the other side of the garden. The cannon at three miles from the trenches sounded pretty loud to me, but no one seemed in the least concerned. The officers chatted over their refreshments and asked me questions about the American Ambulance. I heard two officers having an animated discussion and thought that it must be news of a German attack ahead of us, or at least an account of a trench raid. When I listened to what they said I was relieved and perhaps disappointed to learn that they were discussing the merits of an aria of a recent opera!

In one of Gouverneur Morris' writings he brings out the attitude of the French soldiers to danger as illustrated by Dumas' famous character Athos. He may be excitable over the ordinary episodes of life, but when real danger comes his nerves are like cold steel. And so it seemed to me on my visit to the front. The expressed vivacity of the commonplace existence is replaced by a calmness and determination of spirit as danger is approached. It seemed as if every man from the day he was mobilized had devoted his life to his country and every day that he was spared meant one more day of grace. If death came, as it surely would to many of them, it would find them calm and ready.

After thanking our host for his hospitality, we climbed into another automobile which was protected to the extent of being roofed over and covered in on all sides with little windows in the walls. As we passed out of Suippes it was reassuring to see the peasants gathering their crops within shell-fire range. The road now ran straight as a die for the North. The roadway, partly lined with trees, some of them smashed by shells, was narrow and deserted. Between the tree trunks wires had been strung and interwoven with cut branches which partially hid from the enemy's vision any body of troops or vehicles. My eyes were glued to the little window and what I could see through the narrow aperture and through rifts in the protective barriers of branches looked something like this :

The great plain of Champagne stretched out before us. On the left the mountains of Rheims appeared in the distance. On the right the plateau stretched off into space as far as the eye could see. The country was almost flat. There were low rises of ground, hardly to be called hills. There was not a sign of a living thing except for one weary looking poilu, who was resting with his back against a tree along the wayside. Not a house or a tree was standing in the distance. The whole country looked as if it had been clawed by some immense giant in his rage. There were lines of trenches running in bewildering directions, barbed wire entanglements, great shell-holes. A little grass grew here and there—the rest was the grayish white clay of Champagne. Our car lost no time in covering the three miles, and before I realized where we were, we passed through the ruined village of Souain and stopped behind a protecting bank. Right at hand in the bank was a doorway and stairs leading to a "Poste de Secours." The Médecin-Chef received us and proudly showed us his subterranean hospital. It was more than a dressing station. It was a hospital where badly wounded men, especially abdominal cases, could be operated on right away without the damage of transportation and loss of precious time. The Major had a right to be proud of his institution, as it was splendid in every way. Deep in the earth, well protected from shells, were a series of corridors with rooms leading off from them with cement floors, walls of wood lined with tin painted white, and lighted by electricity and acetylene gas. There were operating rooms, X-ray room, wards for patients, kitchen and store rooms, all complete. Here the wounded are carried, walk or crawl from the firing trench by connecting trenches called "boyaux." Wounded that can be transported are sent to the rear by night in automobiles over the same road we had come. Dinner was being cooked when we arrived. The stove was large and burned charcoal, the fumes making their exit by a pipe leading through the roof and ending at the ground level. Charcoal gives no smoke and tells no tales. The night before as they were finishing some of the construction, two shells dropped near the entrance, the noise of the hammers having indicated the position sufficiently.

A fine spring of clear water was within easy reach of the entrance. Towards the rear was all that was left of the village of Souain. It was simply a disordered mass of stones in hopeless confusion, a relic of the great offensive in September, 1915.

When we climbed up on top of the bank along side the entrance and looked ahead we saw, 1200 metres away, a curving white line extending across the crest of a little rise in a wavy outline. This was the first line of German trenches. The French first line, nearer to us, showed the same white curved line—white because all the soil is a whitish clay. The "boyaux," also curving, led down to our station. As far as the eye could see the terrain was hopelessly clawed by pick and shovel and torn by shell explosions. A few stumps of trees remained here and there. There were booms of cannon at irregular intervals—French 75 and 105 and German 105. It was fascinating and thrilling. The day was bright and clear without a breath of air stirring, and between the cannon shots there was a death-like silence. One knew that within the range of vision there were thousands of men standing in those lines of trenches extended before us and which stretched over 500 miles long from the Swiss frontier to the North Sea. Yet there was not a sign of life movement, and had it not been for the unceasing explosions of the cannon one might have had the same feeling of solitude as when looking over the barren old lava flows of Hawaii. The artillery, so carefully hidden that it could not be seen at all, added to the mystery of it all. The earth and rocks thrown into the air by the shell explosions was the only sign of movement. As we looked out at the scene which to me was most fascinating and thought-producing, a cannon suddenly banged— it seemed right behind us. I looked around and could see nothing but the ruined village. They told me it was a soixante-quinze hidden in the ruins, but there was nothing to be seen of men, cannon or smoke. It seemed like a polite invitation to get down which we did at once. Just then the German cannon started up furiously with a different tone. "They are shooting at an aeroplane," said an officer without looking up. Sure enough, away up over the lines, was a French aeroplane with shells bursting around it. It seemed as if it must be struck, but it was not and sailed majestically back to the rear.

It had come time to depart but I did not want to leave. I was fascinated and at the same time bewildered. I wanted more time to take it all in and comprehend it. This was War as I had never seen it. For a year in hospitals I had cared for wounded, torn by shells and bullets, but here was where men were killed and lay unburied and rotted in the sunshine. A magnificent test of courage to stand up and face the foe with shells bursting and death hovering everywhere, but why should there be war? A curse on those who were responsible for it!

We thanked our host, climbed into our car and went back by the road we had come, past the ruined village, past the poilu still resting with his back against a tree. My eyes were glued to the small window as I looked out on the vast scene of desolation and thought of the brave boys lined up there in the trenches and of their mothers, wives and sweethearts anxious in their homes throughout the land. War seemed an unholy and wicked thing to me.

The sound of the cannon gradually became dimmer until as we approached Châlons we could hear it no more and our visit to the trenches was only a very vivid memory.

CHAPTER XIX.

LEAVING FRANCE AND HOME AGAIN.

After a year's work among the wounded we came to feel very much as if we belonged there. Neutrality was only a form laid out by governmental decree. We were heart and soul with France in her struggle. Consequently the time of departure was a sad one. The night before we were to leave, we were called into one of the wards where all of the blessés who could move or be moved had assembled as well as the staff. At the end of the ward was a table draped with a French flag on which reposed a beautiful large silver cup and a bunch of roses. We were escorted down the ward to our seats at the table to the accompaniment of much handclapping. As soon as we were seated a sergeant read this speech so full of delicate French expression.

Monsieur le Médecin-Chef.

C'est le coeur serré,, que ce soir, je me permets de prendre la parole, au nom de mes camarades, pour vous faire nos adieux. Et pourtant, cher Docteur, je n'ai, ni la capacité nécessaire, ni les qualités d'un orateur, pour vous exprimer comme je le voudrais, comme je le ressens: notre reconnaissance.

Voici plus d'un an, que vous avez quitté votre patrie, votre maison, vos intérêts et que vous avez traversé les océans pour nous apporter vos soins éclairés. Rien ne vous y obligeait: Neutre, vous pouviez suivre le conflit, d'un oeil lointain. Mais votre conscience vous a indiqué un devoir plus haut et vous avez voulu payer de votre personne.

Quel joli geste! Aussi, Docteur, combien nous vous admirons.

Pendant un an, vous vous êtes penché sur nos souffrances, vous êtes intervenu pour les guérir. Combien d'entre ceux qui sont passés ici, vous doivent la vie!

En même temps, placé à la tête de cette importante formation, vous lui donniez une impulsion nouvelle et vous lui faisiez atteindre son rendement maximum.

L'Ambulance Américaine de Juilly a été pour nous une grande famille. Aussi, à côté des impressions horribles de cette guerre, qui ensanglante presque l'Europe entière garderons nous, de notre séjour près de vous, un souvenir très doux et ineffaçable.

Je ne voudrais point terminer sans exprimer à Madame Judd tout notre reconnaissance. Par ses bonnes paroles et son charme, Madame Judd savait nous réconforter, nous faisant oublier nos souffrances, physiques et morales.

Permettez-moi, Docteur, de vous offrir ce souvenir, au nom de tous.

C'est peu, en comparaison de ce que vous avez fait pour nous. Puisse-t-il, vous rappeler quelques fois, vos petits blessés de Juilly.

Dans quelques jours, cher Docteur, vous serez de l'autre côté le l'océan, mais soyez persuadé, que jamais nous ne vous oublierons et souvent notre coeur ira vous rejoindre dans cette Amérique que nous ne connaissons pas, mais que nous avons appris à aimer.

Vive l'Amérique.

Vive La France.

He then presented us with the loving cup and roses. It was then my turn, but with such a lump in my throat, it would have been difficult to have responded in my native tongue. I got through it some way and tried to tell the three hundred French people present that America had not forgotten what Lafayette and his comrades had done for us in our dark days, that victory would come for the side of right and that France would fight on, as she had in the past, until the invader was driven out.

That we had come from the far-off islands of the Pacific to show our sympathy for the cause of France and to work for her brave wounded soldiers. Now that it had come time for us to depart we would carry with us priceless memories of our friends, the poilus.

During our last few hours at the ambulance we made our farewell call on the Mayor, and then shook hands and said goodbye to every one of the poilus. As many as could accompanied us to the doorway where, as we entered our automobile, a farewell cheer was given us. There were tears too in many an eye and our eyes were not dry. We felt as if we were leaving a home and dear friends in a great struggle.

It is easier to get out of France than to enter it. Our American passports were viséd at the consulate, then at the Prefecture of Police our "permis de séjour" were taken up and permission to depart was authorized on our passports. There remained the trip to Bordeaux, with its charming views of the Loire valley, Cathedral of Orleans, Châteaux of Blois and Amboise.

About the only sign of war were husky, well-fed German prisoners working along the railway. At Bordeaux the passports had to be again stamped and we bade farewell to good French cooking by a dinner at the famous "Chapon Fin."

The "Lafayette" lay at a quai piled high with an endless amount of freight from America. We pulled out at midnight and by daybreak we were at the mouth of the Garonne and plunged at once into the swell of the Bay of Biscay. The green shores of France gradually faded away in the distance. No destroyers accompanied us. Our good ship's speed and the rough waters were our best protection. The ship was crowded and there were some famous people aboard. It was not a gay crowd and even the usual concert was omitted. Life preservers were kept handy and there was a general feeling of relief after the second day of our voyage was ended successfully. Nothing occurred to mark the trip until the last day out. When we were sitting out on deck in the afternoon we suddenly noticed that the sun, which had been shining in our faces, now shone over our shoulders. Looking astern we could see a wide curved streak made by the change in our course. At once rumors flew about the ship—"The Kronprinzessin Cecelie had escaped and was after us." "A woman passenger had received a wireless telling her to wear her life-preserver day and night." "A submarine had been sighted," etc. No information could be obtained from the officers. They maintained their usual imperturbability. The look-out men in the crow's nest were relieved frequently. The gun crew were constantly on the watch. We could not believe that danger threatened us right off our home port. There was nothing to do that night but go to bed with a feeling of uncertainty.

Early the next morning we were off Sandy Hook. When the pilot came aboard we learned then for the first time of the depredations of the U-53, of the torpedoing of passenger ships off our coast and of the rescue of women and children from the icy waters. We were thankful to have escaped a similar fate.

The city was hidden in a blanket of fog so that not even the unique sky line of the "scrapers" could be seen. The custom house examination is usually as disagreeable as officiousness and lack of courtesy can make it and this trip was no exception.

It was rather early in the morning and not one familiar face was to be seen on the dock. We were soon plunged into the roar of New York. How different everything seemed! There were no uniforms on the street and there were so many men! Everyone was hurrying about his business and the war might have been on another planet.

At night Broadway was ablaze with lights, with gay restaurants filled with people eating long course dinners. The hotels were turning away people and visitors had to seek accommodations in Jersey City or Brooklyn. Theatres and cabarets were jammed with gay and thoughtless crowds. Money was being spent like water. Much of this money was war profits—the tears and agony of Europe. I heard a well informed person say "The United States has made $20 per capita out of the war and has given less than 35 cents to France and Belgium."

Years of lack of education in our history and ideals combined with apathy and careless living had done its work.

The American people as a whole little realized the purposes of the war and the gravity of the situation. The idea that the Allies were fighting our war, for our principles of liberty and humanity and that America was imperilled by Germany's lust for world conquest had entered the heads of a very small proportion of our fellow citizens. Instead of that the active propaganda for the German language and "Kultur" in our schools, colleges and legislatures, combined with the activities of the German press and German organizations, had weakened the development of a national opposition to Germany's plan of world-empire. The pulpits were woefully deficient in presenting to the people the moral issues of the war, some pulpits even preaching a spirit of "peace at any price." Public writers, teachers and professors neglected their opportunity of bringing to the minds of America what the tragedy of Europe meant.

There were some brave spirits who kept America's soul burning as Theodore Roosevelt, Lyman Abbot, George H. Putnam and James M. Beck, and noble women in different parts of the land were working for the suffering humanity of Europe. The 50,000 or so Americans in the British Army, the Americans in the Foreign Legion, the American aviators, the Ambulance drivers, doctors and nurses all helped to keep

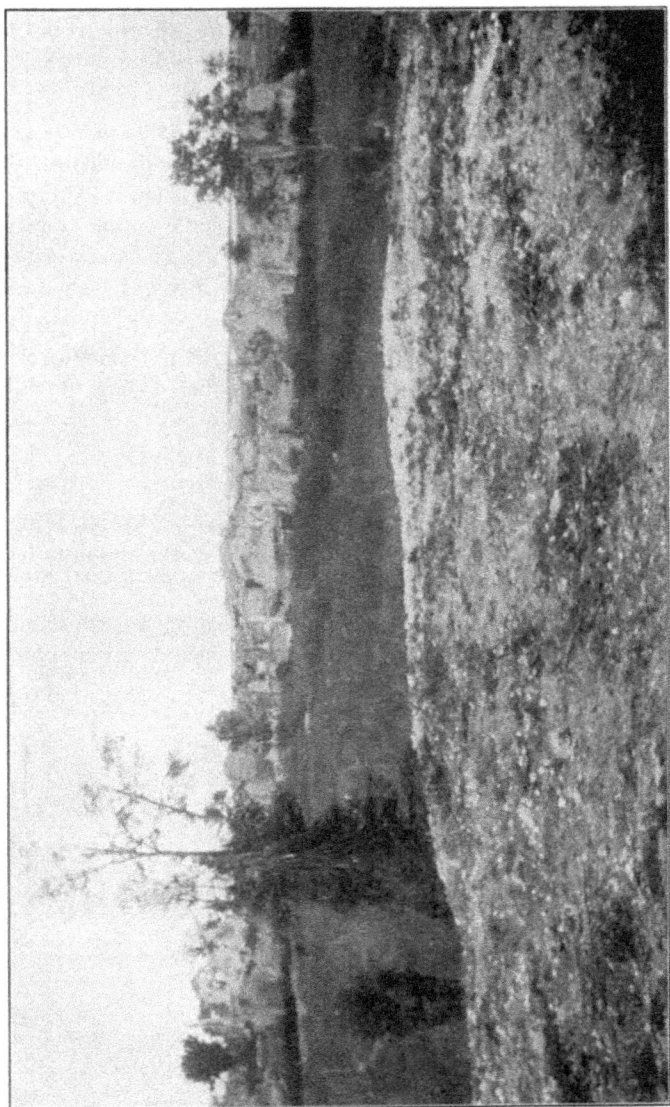

The ruined village of Souain.

alive in France a friendly feeling for the United States and bring closer to our people the cause they tried to serve.

We could not get used to the indifference and smug self-satisfaction in the atmosphere. Will America never wake up? Well, perhaps she will when more Americans are murdered on the seas by the pirate's submarines, and more of our rights are trampled on.

I listened impatiently one evening to a long argument of an eloquent young minister against military training. The gist of his argument was that we should not fight until we were attacked and then all the men could be called on. He failed to bring out what a happy slaughter these unprepared defenders would make for the Huns. The Pacifists at 3,000 miles away from the trenches talked glibly about peace on earth, but when it was proposed to them, none of them relished the idea of having their children spitted on a Prussian bayonet.

During several months in the East I spent some time raising money for ambulances. I found the Americans generous when the good work that our boys were doing at the front was brought to their attention. There was a woeful lack of understanding of the situation. If the American people were not ready to go into the war, it was largely because the facts had not been properly presented to them.

If the realization of what the war meant was feeble in New York, it faded away as one went West, until on the Pacific coast we found that the war was almost an unusual topic of conversation.

Again embarked on the ocean, this time with no fear of German submarines, we sailed the Pacific until our beloved islands came in sight and we were home again.